Artificial Intelligence for Improved Patient Outcomes

Principles for Moving Forward with Rigorous Science

Artificial Intelligence for Improved Patient Outcomes

Principles for Moving Forward with Rigorous Science

Daniel W. Byrne, MS

*Director of Artificial Intelligence Research
Advanced Vanderbilt Artificial Intelligence Laboratory
Departments of Biostatistics, Medicine, and Biomedical Informatics
Vanderbilt University Medical Center
Nashville, Tennessee*

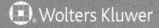

Philadelphia · Baltimore · New York · London
Buenos Aires · Hong Kong · Sydney · Tokyo

Acquisitions Editor: Joe Cho
Development Editors: Anne Malcolm and Dave Murphy
Editorial Coordinator: Priyanka Alagar
Marketing Manager: Kirstin Watrud
Production Project Manager: Bridgett Dougherty
Manager of Graphic Arts and Design: Steve Druding
Manufacturing Coordinator: Beth Welsh
Prepress Vendor: TNQ Technologies

9   8   7   6   5   4   3   2   1

Printed in the United States of America

Library of Congress Cataloging-in-Publication Data

ISBN-13: 978-1-975197-93-3

Cataloging in Publication data available on request from publisher.

shop.LWW.com

MPP1221

For my brilliant wife Loretta, whose thoughtful edits and contributions made this book possible.

—Daniel W. Byrne

The timing is ideal for AI in medicine to improve patient health outcomes. As a result of the convergence of three advances—powerful computers, sophisticated AI algorithms, and comprehensive electronic health records—billions of dollars have been invested in this endeavor. So, this begs the question: *Why is there a dearth of evidence that AI results in improved health for patients?*

The answer lies in the fact that both AI and health care are infinitely complex, abstruse worlds and therefore successfully integrating even a small aspect of these fields requires a deep and mature understanding of what AI can do and what health care needs. Equally important is understanding what AI cannot do and what health care does not need. Much of the slow progress can be attributed to misunderstandings. AI experts have misunderstandings about the problems in health care and health care professionals have misunderstandings about the solutions that AI tools can provide. Progress has been further slowed by health care's fragmented structure and resistance to change.

As a biostatistician working at the intersection of these fields for nearly 40 years, it became clear to me that true success in this unique area requires following fundamental scientific and statistical principles. In this book, we will see that these principles can help overcome the many challenges and improve important patient outcomes. Since one book cannot explain everything about the complex and fast-moving area of AI in medicine, resources for more information are provided at the end of each chapter and in the last chapter.

Special thanks to Henry Domenico, a brilliant biostatistician who built many of the models described in this book, created a number of the key figures, and authored the "*Domenico Guidelines.*" Thanks to Shannon Walker who graciously allowed me to use several of the figures from her *Pediatrics* paper in this book. Shannon is a star physician-scientist who was the PI of the CLOT trial and provided us with a success story to showcase. I am grateful to Ryan Moore, a talented biostatistician and machine learning expert, who made substantial contributions to the content of the book and has been a valuable member of our AVAIL (Advanced Vanderbilt Artificial Intelligence Laboratory) team.

At Vanderbilt University Medical Center, I am fortunate to be part of many successful research teams who conducted these projects and made fundamental advances in AI in medicine. These include Li Wang, Warren Sandberg, Ben French, Laura Beth Brown, Ryan Starnes, Jonathan Grande, Matt Semler, Allison Wheeler, Yu Shyr, C. Michael Stein, Mary Yarbrough, Sreenivasa Balla, Rob Freundlich, Peter Shave, Tony Hernandez, Kevin Patel, Elizabeth Phillips, April Barnardo, Holly Ende, Peg Duthie, Benjamin Tillman, Prince Kannankeril, Kevin Johnson, and Art Wheeler. I am grateful to the members of AVAIL for their insights and support.

Thanks to my family for proofreading, especially Virginia Byrne, Bill Byrne, and Jim Byrne. Thanks to the editors at Wolters-Kluwer: Acquisitions Editor, Joe Cho, Development Editor, Thomas Celona, Development Editor, Dave Murphy, and Editorial Coordinator, Priyanka Alagar. I will always be grateful to Elizabeth Nieginski, former Executive Acquisitions Editor for Wolters-Kluwer, for publishing my first book. Most of all, I am grateful to my wonderful wife, Loretta Byrne, for her patience, sharp critical eye, and insightful editing of this book.

Contents

Daniel Byrne is a biostatistician and Artificial Intelligence investigator at Vanderbilt University with 40 years of experience at the leading edge of AI implementation in health care. In his role as Director of Artificial Intelligence Research for AVAIL (Advanced Vanderbilt Artificial Intelligence Laboratory) he builds and tests AI models in pragmatic randomized controlled trials. Byrne is known for his discoveries on how Artificial Intelligence and predictive models can be integrated into health care and then assessed with scientific rigor to determine whether they improve health outcomes.

As a faculty member in the Department of Biostatistics at Vanderbilt, Byrne has taught graduate-level courses to hundreds of physician-scientists and won numerous teaching awards. He is the author of the award-winning book *Publishing Your Medical Research* and more than 150 medical research papers, including landmark pragmatic trials, which have appeared in journals such as *The New England Journal of Medicine*, *JAMA*, and *The Lancet*.

For more information, see vumc.org/biostatistics/person/daniel-w-byrne

The Big Picture

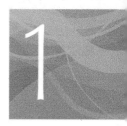

Overview—How Artificial Intelligence Will Improve Health

The improvement of patient health outcomes is the primary objective of Artificial Intelligence (AI) in health care. All other advantages that may result thereafter are secondary. The information provided in this book demonstrates how AI has been applied to predict outcomes, support decision making, and prevent errors. Yet in some ways AI has started off on the wrong foot and therefore has a tarnished reputation. This technology is still relatively new to health care and ironically has been presented by some as a "cure all" or a "quick fix" to complex problems. This combination of events has resulted in a general mistrust of AI. The goal of this book is to demonstrate and encourage AI and medical professionals to build wisely, implement carefully, and recognize the mistrust and overcome it with rigorous science.

Medicine is the area of society in which AI will have the most positive impact, but unfortunately it still lags far behind other industries. The following chapters describe why medicine is so far behind and provide an optimistic, yet practical, transformational playbook for moving forward.

PRINCIPLE 1 • Improving patient health is the primary goal of AI in medicine. Secondary goals can include lowering costs and reducing the burden on clinicians.

When implemented properly, the value-added proposition of AI is that the quality of patient outcomes will improve, justifying the costs, and the cost will be reduced over time due to AI's impact. Although AI will only be one part of the solution for improving health care, Table 1.1 lists potential ways AI will add value, with value defined as:

$$\text{Value} = \frac{\text{Quality}}{\text{Cost}}$$

TABLE 1.1	Potential Ways AI Could Help Improve the Health Care System

Improved Patient Safety

Focused prevention

Reduced unwarranted variation in clinical practice

Improved accuracy of interpretation of medical images

Reduced adverse drug events and avoidable medical errors

Reduced deaths from preventable errors

Improved precision and speed of prognoses

Improved patient handoffs in care settings with efficient transfer of information

Improved patient experience and satisfaction

Improved Clinician Decision Support

Identification of disease subtypes that respond differently to treatments

Improved diagnostic precision, reducing diagnostic errors

Efficient time to diagnosis

Optimized timing of evidence-based treatment

Precision/personalized medicine becomes a reality—moving from one-size-fits-all

Improved Equity and Fairness

Reduced health inequities and health disparities

Reduced racial biases

Empowered patient autonomy

Improved Work Environment for Clinicians

Reduced information overload with useful decision support and actionable choices

Specialist-level decision support in areas with too few specialists

Health care providers will have time to make health care human again[1]

Clinicians will have time to be empathetic (56% do not have time for this now)

Reduced clinician burnout, now estimated at 35%

TABLE 1.1	*Continued*

Improved Efficiency

Cost reduction (one-third of current health care spending in the United States is waste)[1,2]

Improved triage systems

Reduced costs to patients by reducing waste and reducing insurance denials

Reduced medical malpractice by improving patient safety

Improved efficiency of patient throughput and hospital capacity management

PRINCIPLE 2 • Use a broad and inclusive definition of AI.

Let's define AI. The late computer scientist, Larry Tesler had this sarcastic definition:

> *"AI is whatever hasn't been done yet."*
>
> —Tesler's Theorem

We will define AI as the development of computer systems and mathematical models that mimic cognitive functions (that humans associate with the human mind) and that perform tasks that normally require human intelligence. These tasks include prediction, object detection, speech recognition, learning, decision making, and solving complex problems such as risk stratification. AI will be defined very broadly in this book to include not only machine learning, neural networks, deep learning, but also traditional statistical techniques for creating predictive models, such as logistic regression (Figure 1.1).

Hours can be spent debating the definition of AI, but instead we will skip this debate and use a broad definition of AI to move forward focusing on accomplishing something important. In fact, one of the reasons that health care is lagging so far behind in AI applications is this Brownian motion of academics in medical centers engaging in endless debates over definitions rather than advancing forward. At the other extreme from academia, many in the AI industry push the implementation of AI faster than appropriate and skip important discussions and steps necessary for successful implementation

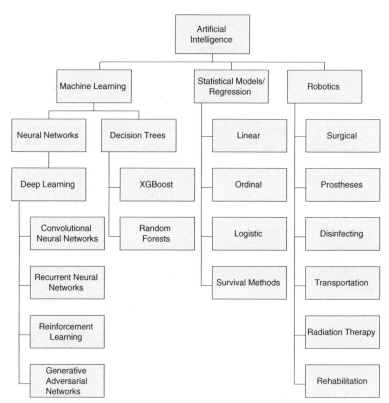

FIGURE 1.1. Categories of Artificial Intelligence. The major branches of AI are machine learning, statistical regression predictive models, and robotics. Regression is then categorized by the level of measurement for the outcome: continuous (linear regression), ordinal (ordinal regression), binary (logistic regression), and censored, time-to-event (survival methods). Machine learning can be divided into decision trees and neural networks, with deep learning as a subset of neural networks. Within deep learning, there are important subgroups: convolutional neural networks, recurrent neural networks, reinforcement learning, and generative adversarial networks.

and evaluations. The term Artificial Intelligence is not ideal, but it is too late to change it. Some have tried to rebrand AI as Augmented Intelligence or Cognitive Computing, which are more accurate, but neither term has been widely adopted. Success will require finding the sweet spot by combining the best of both Industry and Academia—while minimizing the weaknesses and baggage of each side (Figure 1.2).

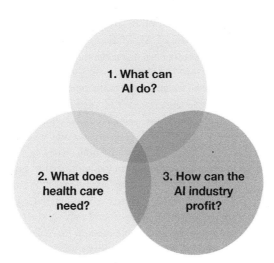

FIGURE 1.2. Venn diagram of three key questions. Forward progress will require that we understand the answers to these questions and focus on the appropriate areas of overlap. Health care systems that wish to partner with AI vendors need to find projects at the intersection of the circles. Physician-scientists have a larger space to find successful projects that are in the intersection of questions 1 and 2.

PRINCIPLE 3 • Create academic-industry synergy.

The U.S. health care system is full of many smart, hardworking, wonderful people who are doing their best to care for and cure patients, yet the system they are working within has misaligned incentives.[2] While AI can help fix this system, most health care organizations are struggling to execute AI. Overcoming this requires that we identify and recognize how previous AI tools for medicine failed and solve these problems with modern reproducible research.

One fear or obstacle to overcome is the myth that implementation with randomized trials of AI will be expensive, lengthy, multicentered, and too difficult to conduct. As we will see from the examples in this book, this is untrue. Few people in the AI or medical community understand why this randomization is vital and how it can be accomplished in an ethical, rapid, and pragmatic way. Academic scientists and clinicians understand the need for randomization, but it is new to others. Fostering an environment which incentivizes testing approaches in a low-cost manner creates a synergy to move forward.

Scientists must take the lead in evaluating the effectiveness and impact of AI. Marketing and salespeople must limit their claims to scientifically valid and published conclusions.

In the past, aggressive marketing of the benefits of AI in medicine has hindered the progress and use of AI. Marketing teams, sales groups, vendors, advertisers, and the media have made claims that were sometimes: (1) not true, (2) exaggerated, or (3) did not present the information on clinical impact in a way that allowed for an honest evaluation. Health care executives, hospital administrators, and clinicians often lacked the skills and knowledge to make rational decisions about purchasing AI tools being pitched. This mismatch led to poor decisions, wasteful investments, and resentment. Today, senior health care executives must have a solid understanding of what AI can and cannot do in health care. Although they do not need to understand the technical details, they must understand the larger issues of AI in medicine.

Only after objective scientists conduct a randomized controlled trial (RCT) testing the impact of each AI tool, and publish the complete findings in a transparent way in a high-profile medical journal, should we trust the claims of these marketing teams. This strategy will be more valuable and effective than any brochure, PowerPoint presentation, or cute advertising campaign that overpromises about pseudo-innovation.

PRINCIPLE 4 • Recognize that the U.S. health care system is financially unsustainable but that many of the problems can be solved with carefully implemented and rigorously evaluated AI.

To be clear, the problem is the system—not the people working in the system. The first step in fixing this system is to be brutally honest and evidence-based about the problems (Table 1.2).

Currently, academic medical centers reward faculty for creating and publishing research papers about new AI models. Given the many challenges, little incentive exists for implementation research demonstrating that the model can improve patient outcomes. As a result, we have thousands of papers published on predictive models and very little evidence that they benefit patients. Most models are never implemented. Many cannot be used. Few are automated into the electronic health record (EHR).

PRINCIPLE 5 • A new and modern approach is needed to successfully use AI to improve health outcomes.

AI systems created for health care must be carefully developed, validated, implemented, and tested. They must be more transparent than in the past when AI tools were only partially described and evaluated. For private companies concerned about transparency of their products and services, methods need to be developed to enable them to make a profit and at the same time

TABLE 1.2	Problems in the U.S. Health Care System

Skyrocketing costs

Clinician burnout

Misaligned financial and career incentives

Slow rate of change in adopting new technology and treatments

Reactive downstream diagnoses and treatments

One-size-fits-all approaches rather than personalized medicine

Expensive and clunky electronic health record (EHR) systems

Fee-for-service (quantity is rewarded over quality)

Itemized hospital bills

Medical errors (the third leading cause of death in the United States)[3]

Lack of transparency about costs and outcomes

Lack of true competition

Diagnostic odysseys—excessive time from onset of symptoms to final diagnosis

Only 55% of Americans receive the recommended health care

Disjointed care coordination across the continuum

Outdated and redundant data collection techniques—paper forms on clipboards

More than 100,000 overdose deaths in the past year in the United States

enable scientists to evaluate the impact of the approach. AI tools should be evaluated and validated in a rigorous way on a diverse population to help ensure fairness and equity. The model should be reported in an open way to enable others to reproduce it and compare to alternative approaches. For an example of how to transparently report a model, see: "A Real-time Risk-Prediction Model for Pediatric Venous Thromboembolic Events." [4]

PRINCIPLE 6 • Learn how other industries use AI to improve safety and efficiency.

Comparison of AI's impact between the airline industry and health care

Over a 12-year period (2009-2021), U.S. airlines carried 8 billion passengers without a single fatal crash.[5] During that same period, U.S. hospitals had more than 264,000 preventable deaths.[6] This is the equivalent of 565, 747-jets crashing—or one per week. One of the major reasons for this discrepancy is that the airline industry applies AI and computer modeling routinely and broadly to improve safety while health care does not. The airline industry has successfully implemented AI for weather modeling, autopilot, flight simulators, landing systems, predictive machinery maintenance, black box/flight recorder analyses, and air traffic control systems. The airline industry has integrated these components of technology to provide a pilot-computer synergy, which functions in a frictionless way. While many will be quick to dismiss this comparison by saying that the health care and airline industries are very different, there is no doubt that health care can do better and learn from industries that are much safer and more advanced with cutting-edge technology seamlessly woven into the workflow.

What causes preventable hospital deaths and how could the airline AI approach be used? One of the leading causes of preventable hospital deaths in the United States is a blood clot (venous thromboembolism [VTE]). With the CLOT (Children's Likelihood Of Thrombosis) study, my Vanderbilt colleagues and I have shown that an AI tool can be automated in the EHR to identify these clots before they happen and then the prevention program can be tested in a pragmatic RCT.[4] This example, as well as others, will be used throughout the book to illustrate specific points.

PRINCIPLE 7 • Improving health outcomes requires making better decisions—under uncertainty and in an environment of information overload. These decisions often require making predictions and although AI does not create real intelligence, it does create a component of intelligence: prediction.[7]

> *"Medicine is the science of uncertainty and the art of probability."*
> —Sir William Osler

First, there is no real intelligence with AI. AI cannot critically interpret the medical literature. AI does not understand meaning, reasoning, or cause-effect concepts. AI does not know what to do for high-risk patients. AI will add value, not by pretending that it provides real intelligence, but by using the component of intelligence that it does provide in a manner that benefits clinicians.

Clinical Decision Support Systems

The proper use of AI is as clinical decision support—not clinical decision replacement. In many areas of medicine AI can, or will soon, provide more accurate, cheaper, and faster prediction than humans[7] by combining the best of what computers do with the best of what humans do. Then rigorous science, spearheaded by physician-scientists, will assess if AI improves health, without causing unexpected problems, and without cutting corners.

PRINCIPLE 8 • **AI clinical decision support tools can provide precise and accurate granular risk stratification to reduce heterogeneity that is present within the current staging and risk grouping categories.**

Risk stratification, the process of separating patients by level of care needed, is an important application of AI in medicine. Accurate, automated, and timely risk stratification is needed to improve most measurements in health care. Currently our health care system accepts too much heterogeneity within the staging/risk grouping categories, for example Stage 1 to 4. With our modern tools, we do not need to be limited to the broad groups. In each area of medicine, however, one can witness the slow evolution of risk stratification from none, to dichotomous, to points, to a continuous probability that the outcome will occur—from 0% to 100%.

Personalized medicine and risk stratification

"One-size-fits-all" is obviously a flawed approach for many aspects of health care and yet it is all too common. "Two-sizes-fit-all" is not much of an improvement and yet most of our health care system unnecessarily dichotomizes patients as low- or high-risk. A point scoring system is a step in the right direction and is often seen as innovation—but this is still antiquated and suboptimal. The ideal way to improve many health outcomes is to have evidence-based granular risk stratification automatically displayed as probabilities of outcome based on AI models. AI will transform health care in many ways, but one of the most important will be accurate, timely, inexpensive, and precise risk stratification.

Risk stratification has evolved over time as seen in Figure 1.3. This improvement in risk stratification enables better prediction (Figure 1.4). Using our CLOT study as an example, prevention of blood clots among hospitalized patients (or in medical terminology, prophylaxis for VTE) could be based on no risk stratification, treating all patients the same—either they all

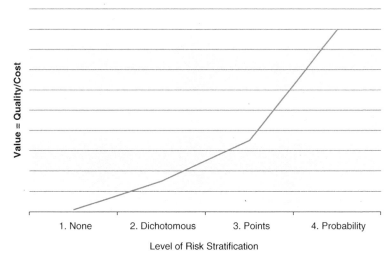

FIGURE 1.3. Evolution of risk stratification and value. As areas of health care move to more advanced, evidence-based, and granular levels of risk stratification, outcomes will improve and costs will decrease, leading to increased value. This cartoon illustrates the general relationship of risk stratification and value. For many medical interventions, without risk stratification, there is no value. Categorizing patients as high risk or low risk provides a slight improvement in value. Using a point scoring system to create a scale provides better risk stratification and value. The ultimate level of risk stratification is from an accurate and precise predictive model that provides a probability of the outcome from 0% to 100%.

receive prophylaxis, or none do. Obviously, this is not optimal. Patients could be divided into low-risk or high-risk, but this is suboptimal. Points could be assigned for risk factors, but this is not completely evidence-based and leaves information on the table for no reason. Alternatively, creating a predictive model of VTE and providing granular evidence-based probabilities of the VTE from 0% to 100% improves the accuracy with which the clinician can predict and improve outcomes.[4]

Figure 1.5 illustrates the problem of allocating limited prevention resources without risk stratification. The high-risk patients did not routinely obtain prevention in a reliable and timely way. At the low-risk extreme patients were receiving prevention resources that were unneeded and sometimes harmful, while with risk stratification, the limited prevention resources were allocated efficiently and effectively. High-risk patients might need one-on-one prevention, the middle group less intense prevention, and the low-risk group no prevention.

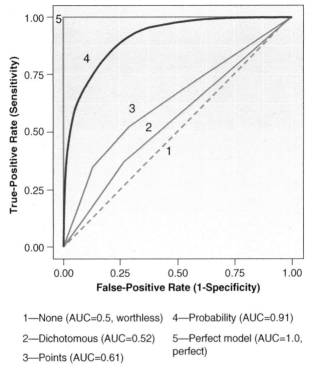

1—None (AUC=0.5, worthless) 4—Probability (AUC=0.91)

2—Dichotomous (AUC=0.52) 5—Perfect model (AUC=1.0, perfect)

3—Points (AUC=0.61)

FIGURE 1.4. Evolution of risk stratification and accuracy of predictions. This receiver-operating-characteristics curve demonstrates the increased accuracy of predictive models based on the level of predictor stratification. This graph plots the specificity versus the sensitivity for the various points from a predictive model. For example, if the model predicts that a patient has 91% risk of a complication, the sensitivity might be 80% and the specificity might be 90%. The area under the receiver-operating-characteristic curve (AUC) is a measure of the model's performance. A completely worthless predictive model, which is no better than flipping a coin, has an AUC of 0.5. A perfect model has an AUC of 1.0. As areas of health care move to more sophisticated levels of risk stratification, the predictions become more accurate. (Reproduced with permission from Pediatrics, Walker SC, Creech CB, Domenico HJ, French B, Byrne DW, Wheeler AP. A real-time risk-prediction model for pediatric venous thromboembolic events. *Pediatrics.* 2021;147(6):e2020042325. Copyright © 2020 by the AAP.)

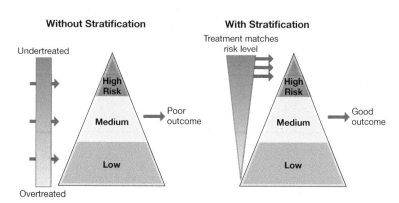

FIGURE 1.5. Risk stratification is essential for focused prevention and treatment. Many health care interventions fail to improve outcome unless an accurate, timely, and granular risk stratification can focus limited prevention and treatment resources where they are most needed. Without this stratification, resources are spread across risk levels. With risk stratification, resources are focused on the high risk, leading to better outcomes.

A common problem in risk stratification that should be avoided is the practice of converting most continuous predictor and outcome variables into two categories, which is known as "dichotomania."[8,9] This is common when the user has limited experience and skill in working with continuous variables. For example, body mass index (BMI) can be used to predict type 2 diabetes. One could use the continuous BMI or dichotomize into obese or not (BMI ≤ 30 or >30). Figure 1.6 illustrates the information loss caused by dichotomizing. The efficiency of dichotomizing a continuous variable can be estimated as $1\text{-}(2/\text{pi})$, which would require studying 1580 patients with a dichotomous predictor versus 1000 with a continuous predictor.

Obviously, one-size-fits-all would be a fiasco for many areas of health care, for example, blood transfusions or prescription glasses. For more complex stratification problems, AI tools can guide clinical practice and help move forward out of the all-or-none world.

PRINCIPLE 9 • A pragmatic randomized controlled trial is the key to real progress of AI in health care.

The hyperbole, the claims based on weak evaluations with slick marketing slogans, has successfully raised interest and funding in AI (Figure 1.7). But, to date, we have little evidence of improvements in health. AI will transform health care in the near future, but before that can happen, rigorous science

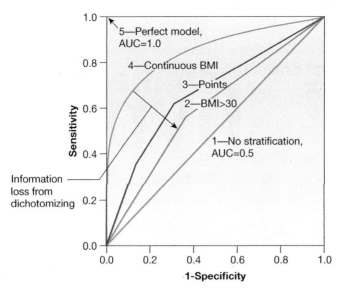

FIGURE 1.6. Impact of dichotomizing a predictor variable. This receiver-operating-characteristics curve illustrates the unnecessary information loss due to dichotomizing body mass index (BMI). 1—no risk stratification results in a worthless model with an area under the receiver-operating-characteristic curve (AUC) of 0.5. 2—dichotomizing the BMI (≤30 versus >30) results in a poor model. 3—a point scoring system (0: ≤25, 1: 25-27.5, 2: 27.5-29.9, 3: 30-34.9, 4: ≥35) results in a slightly better model. 4—using the continuous BMI provides the best model. 5—a perfect predictive model would reach the upper left corner with an AUC of 1.0.

is needed to learn how to best implement these tools. Specifically, medicine needs adaptive platform prospective patient-level RCTs that assess important health outcomes, which are published in peer-reviewed, high-profile medical journals. These trials (described in Chapter 9) can be designed as low-cost pragmatic trials.

Implementation of AI must be compared with current usual medical care. These comparisons must assess real-world evaluations for effectiveness, harm, and unintended consequences. The subject of randomization is so important, misunderstood, and complex that the entire Chapter 2 is devoted to the topic of AI randomization. Most AI research has been limited to nonrandomized, retrospective, observational studies, or weak study designs, such as before-after (historical controls). This must change to fix the "AI chasm," which refers to the gap between a model's statistical performance and improving what matters to patients.[10,11]

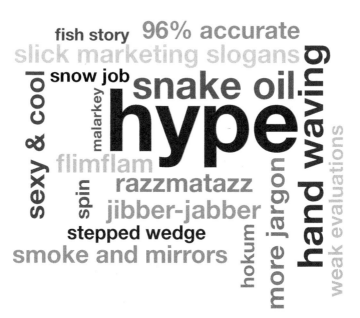

FIGURE 1.7. Word cloud of AI hyperbole. What is missing in this word cloud is "pragmatic randomized controlled trial."

These studies must raise the current level of evaluation and follow the modern reporting standards and recommendations. These can be found in the following documents: TRIPOD—"Transparent Reporting of a multivariable prediction model for Individual Prognosis Or Diagnosis,"[12] and TRIPOD-AI.[13] Also see: "Reporting guidelines for clinical trial reports for interventions involving artificial intelligence: the CONSORT-AI Extension."[14,15] In addition to the 37 items in the CONSORT checklist, 14 additional items are specific to AI projects.

---

i **FOR MORE INFORMATION**

Deep Medicine: How Artificial Intelligence Can Make Healthcare Human Again. Eric Topol.[1]
Welcoming new guidelines for AI clinical research. Eric Topol.[16]
How AI Can Promote Accuracy and Medicine. Eric Topol.[17]

CHAPTER SUMMARY

Artificial Intelligence will be used to add value by improving health outcomes and lowering costs—but until now we have seen more exaggeration than evidence.[1] The proper incentives are needed to both raise the level of rigor and change the focus to patient-centric end points. AI tools need to be evaluated and validated on large, diverse populations to assess fairness and equity. The models should be reported in an open way to enable others to reproduce them and compare alternative approaches. Most health care organizations are struggling to execute AI. Overcoming this requires identifying and recognizing how previous AI implementation for medicine failed and solve these problems with modern reproducible research.

REFERENCES

1. Topol E. *Deep Medicine: How Artificial Intelligence Can Make Healthcare Human Again.* Basic Books; 2019.
2. Spellberg B. *Broken, Bankrupt, and Dying: How to Solve the Great American Healthcare Rip-off.* Lioncrest Publishing; 2020.
3. Makary MA, Daniel M. Medical error-the third leading cause of death in the US. *BMJ.* 2016;353:i2139.
4. Walker SC, Creech CB, Domenico HJ, French B, Byrne DW, Wheeler AP. A real-time risk-prediction model for pediatric venous thromboembolic events. *Pediatrics.* 2021;147(6):e2020042325.
5. Pasztor A. The Airline Safety Revolution. *Wall Street Journal.* April 16, 2021. https://www.wsj.com/articles/the-airline-safety-revolution-11618585543
6. Rodwin BA, Bilan VP, Merchant NB, et al. Rate of preventable mortality in hospitalized patients: a systematic review and meta-analysis. *J Gen Intern Med.* 2020;35(7):2099-2106.
7. Agrawal A, Gans J, Goldfarb A. *Prediction Machines: The Simple Economics of Artificial Intelligence.* Harvard Business Review Press; 2018.
8. Senn S. *Dichotomania: An Obsessive Compulsive Disorder that is Badly Affecting the Quality of Analysis of Pharmaceutical Trials.* Semantic scholar; 2005. https://www.isi-web.org/isi.cbs.nl/iamamember/CD6-Sydney2005/ISI2005_Papers/398.pdf
9. Royston P, Altman DG, Sauerbrei W. Dichotomizing continuous predictors in multiple regression: a bad idea. *Stat Med.* 2006;25(1):127-141.
10. Keane PA, Topol EJ. With an eye to AI and autonomous diagnosis. *NPJ Digit Med.* 2018;1:40.
11. Shah NH, Milstein A, Bagley SC. Making machine learning models clinically useful. *J Am Med Assoc.* 2019;322(14):1351-1352.

12. Collins GS, Reitsma JB, Altman DG, et al. Transparent Reporting of a Multivariable Prediction Model for Individual Prognosis or Diagnosis (TRIPOD). *Circulation.* 2015;131:211-219.

13. Collins GS, Moons KGM. Reporting of artificial intelligence prediction models. *Lancet.* 2019;393:1577-1579.

14. Liu X, Rivera SC, Moher D, Calvert MJ, Denniston AK; SPIRIT-AI, CONSORT-AI Working Group. Reporting guidelines for clinical trial reports for interventions involving artificial intelligence: the CONSORT-AI Extension. *BMJ.* 2020;370:m3164.

15. Liu X, Cruz Rivera S, Moher D, Calvert MJ, Denniston AK. Reporting guidelines for clinical trial reports for interventions involving artificial intelligence: the CONSORT-AI extension. *Nat Med.* 2020;26:1364-1374.

16. Topol EJ. Welcoming new guidelines for AI clinical research. *Nat Med.* 2020;26(9):1318-1320.

17. Topol EJ. *How AI Can Promote Accuracy and Empathy in Medicine.* 2021. https://www.youtube.com/watch?v=iclfpf2Gv6Y

Randomization— The "Secret Sauce"

Randomization is not arbitrary or haphazard. In medical research, randomization is the process by which participants in clinical trials are assigned based on chance alone to separate groups that are given different treatments or interventions. Neither the researcher nor the participant chooses which treatment or intervention the participant will receive. This is a process that is truly random and does not follow a deterministic pattern, such as odd vs even hospital admission dates. Randomization can be created by flipping a coin, using a random number table, or having a computer algorithm generate the random assignment (0 vs 1). In a sufficiently large study, random assignment of patients to a new Artificial Intelligence (AI) tool or a control group of usual care greatly increases the likelihood that the only difference between the groups is the AI tool. This enables us to assess the impact of the intervention on outcome without worrying about other confounding factors that make observational studies treacherous. See Table 10.1 for three examples of how randomization has answered important medical questions in pragmatic trials.

Randomization produces comparable groups and minimizes selection bias. Bias here refers to the systematic error (as opposed to random error) introduced into sampling or testing by selecting or encouraging one outcome over others. For example, clinicians might choose to use the AI tool on healthier patients, which would create a bias that would make it impossible to measure the true impact of AI.

Although patient-level randomization, in rigorous scientific trials, is the key, few people in the AI or medical community understand why randomization is important for assessing AI tools and how it can be accomplished in an ethical, rapid, and pragmatic way. Therefore, this chapter is devoted to this topic.

PRINCIPLE 10 • Understand the essential role of randomization and rigorous science in moving AI forward.

A new approach of implementing AI in medicine is needed, specifically one respectful to and thoughtful about the implementation into the existing workflow, which tests the impact on patients with scientific rigor. Several

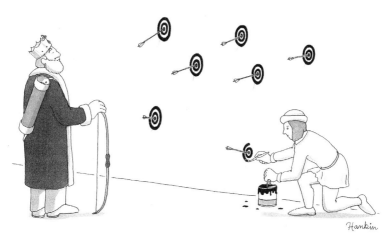

FIGURE 2.1. Pseudo-success. The results in weak evaluations and analyses that are not prespecified are sometimes manipulated to "prove" that AI was successful at improving outcomes [Charlie Hankin/The New Yorker Collection/The Cartoon Bank].

years ago, the chief executive officer of a major hospital was frustrated that patient outcomes were not improving—despite many initiatives to fix them. He said, "I wish I knew what the secret sauce is." **The secret sauce is randomization.**

The assessment of many health care AI interventions is similar to target shooting in the dark. The shooters can claim that they hit the target 100% of the time, but because it is dark, no one knows the truth. By turning on the lights, it is revealed that the shooters were only hitting the target 10% of the time. Like shooting arrows in the dark, when AI tools are introduced into health care without randomization there are often claims of great success. With randomization, we learn the truth. Obviously, resistance will be encountered when moving away from a system that appeared to be successful 100% of the time (Figure 2.1), but randomization shines the light on whether the claims about an AI tool are exaggerated or legitimate and provides the guide toward improvement, allowing for more precision and accuracy.

PRINCIPLE 11 • Recognize invalid ways of assessing AI.

Because AI is new and innovative, it is understandable that there is a desire to push it into current workflows without a rigorous statistical and scientific assessment. But let's look at why this has not been working. Table 2.1 lists

TABLE 2.1	Flawed "Proof" That AI Improves Health Outcomes

Expert testimonials say it works.

A large number of papers have been published in medical journals about the AI tool.

Physicians like it.

An emotional patient testimonial "proves" AI works.

The press release stated that the AI tool is 96% accurate.

It is implemented at many hospitals.

The vendor claims the AI tool:

    detects disease X as well as a doctor.

    has a concordance rate of 94% with physicians-specialists.

    has reached many patients.

    has a sensitivity of 98%!

Our [improperly conducted] stepped wedge study design showed that our AI tool worked.

A poster presented at a medical conference proved that our AI tool worked.

"I do think it improves patient care" one expert said.

some of the invalid methods people have used to "prove" AI works without randomization.

PRINCIPLE 12 • Anticipate fierce and sustained resistance to testing AI with randomization—turning on the lights.

Successful health care and hospital leaders will send the message from the top down that testing AI with randomization and rigorous science is the most important next step toward using this technology. Their message will explain that randomization is necessary to eliminate various types of bias and produce comparable groups needed to establish causal conclusions about AI and outcomes.

Many will be uncomfortable, or object outright, to the use of randomization—anticipate it. Some object in the middle of the utterance of the word "randomization." Therefore, we must understand their objections and concerns and develop solutions that are acceptable to all. Those who object to randomization need to be listened to, but also shown that randomization is essential, and can be conducted in an ethical, low-cost, nimble way that does not cause problems. This is a major mindset shift for many. Those with a traditional, less-rigorous evaluation approach will be most resistant.

Even many of those who now support randomization of AI thought it was unnecessary or wrong earlier in their careers. Experienced biomedical AI researchers have come to realize it is a necessity and that there are ethical ways to conduct randomization. Bioethicists have argued that in many cases, when there is clinical equipoise, it is unethical not to randomize AI tools and thereby lack the information needed to determine cause and effect and avoid unintended consequences.

Proprietary AI models, which do not explain how they work (black boxes), have already been included in commercial electronic health records (EHRs) without randomized evaluations. These are currently used in the care of patients at many hospitals. This approach is problematic and has been criticized.

> *"This external validation cohort study suggests that the ESM [Epic Sepsis Model] has poor discrimination and calibration in predicting the onset of sepsis. The widespread adoption of the ESM despite its poor performance raises fundamental concerns about sepsis management on a national level."*
>
> —WONG ET AL[1]

In his excellent 2019 article titled "Key Challenges for Delivering Clinical Impact with Artificial Intelligence," Christopher Kelly, from Google Health,[2] stated "Robust peer-reviewed clinical evaluation as part of randomized controlled trials should be viewed as the gold standard for evidence generation but conducting these in practice may not always be appropriate or feasible." In this book, we will see how recent advances in pragmatic trials and informatics have made it appropriate and feasible to assess most AI models in randomized controlled trials (RCTs). This type of study is essential to moving beyond statistical metrics of AI models to measures of quality of care and end points that are important to patient well-being.

AI vendors, salespeople, marketing groups, and developers will use a variety of approaches to "show" that their AI tools improve outcome without testing in a randomized trial. Hospital administrators, managers, and clinicians will sometimes also use these methods. Most do not even realize that they are doing something that is fundamentally flawed. Table 2.2 lists the excuses they use to bypass this essential step forward.

TABLE 2.2	Reasons for Refusing to Randomize Impact Studies of AI in Medicine

I. Delays.

Randomizing will slow us down. We are in a rush and just need to fix this and do something fast.

We are putting valuable hospital resources into this intervention.

The end points are important quality metrics with financial penalties [such as 30-day hospital readmissions].

We are in a crisis mode and do not have time for research.

We are under pressure to improve this soon.

Research slows us down!

It is too early to randomize.

It is too late to randomize.

II. Ethics.

Randomization would be unethical.

What if the public found out?

The Institutional Review Board would never allow that.

It will be illegal.

The data are biased.

Just yesterday there was an 80-year-old man who needed X. Are you saying we will withhold that from him?

III. Need.

We already know this works. We just need to implement it.

We aren't going to prove this in a statistical way.

We can just look at the before-after data and use historical controls.

We are not planning on publishing a paper about this. We are not in the business of publishing papers.

Randomized controlled trials (RCTs) will be a barrier to roll out.

You can either prove or improve but you can't do both. So, we are going to improve—and not randomize.

This is Quality Improvement—not research.

We can use observational data and statistically adjust for covariates.

Testing whether this leads to improvements is 5 years down the road. [Note: It is always 5 years down the road.]

Randomization may work in other areas of health care, but our area is special, and it will not work here.

(Continued)

TABLE 2.2   *Continued*

There is already evidence to suggest that this AI tool will reduce morbidity and mortality.

Instead of a randomized controlled trial, we will use a stepped wedge study design. [Note: These often fail to be performed rigorously due to improper randomizing of the clusters, which leads to a flawed conclusion based on regression to the mean.]

There was never a randomized controlled trial for parachutes.

IV. Challenges.

It would be too hard to randomize. Randomization will cause problems.

It would be impossible to display the probability from AI for a random half of the patients in the electronic health record or imaging device.

It would upset the front-line clinical people, such as nurses. Showing a score for half of the patients would cause problems.

We could never get informed written consent from all the patients.

It will upset the boss, CEO of the hospital, dean, etc.

Researchers should pay for this—not hospital operations.

RCTs are impractical and prohibitively expensive.

We do not have the skills to do an RCT.

By recommending randomization, you are not being collaborative.

You cannot randomize everyone in the hospital to information technology or not.

The National Institutes for Health or Centers for Medicare & Medicaid Services will not allow randomization for this project.

The outcome would be too infrequent and the intervention too difficult to detect the impact of AI.

We do not have complete and accurate data on all patients in the electronic health record. [Note: the data will never be 100% complete and accurate, but there are statistical methods that solve the problem of missing data for AI tools.]

"That is not only not right; it is not even wrong!"

—WOLFGANG PAULI, THEORETICAL PHYSICIST, NOBEL
LAUREATE, 1945.

AI needs to be assessed with the scientific method in an RCT in the same way as any new drug or device would be—even if this is not currently required by the U.S. Food and Drug Administration. Anecdotal evidence is meaningless. Larger amounts of anecdotal evidence are not progress. The implementation of AI may be novel, but this alone is not reason to bypass the traditional scientific process.

"The plural of anecdote is not data."

—ATTRIBUTED TO FRANK KOTSONIS, GEORGE STIGLER,
AND ROGER BRINNER.

PRINCIPLE 13 • Understand what was flawed when randomization was not applied.

Lack of randomization often leads to false conclusions. Understand and recognize false assumptions. Let's look at some examples. Imagine if we let clinicians choose whether to use an AI tool on certain patients and then we look at the long-term effects. This approach suffers from "confounding by indication" and therefore has almost no value. Confounding by indication occurs in nonrandomized observational studies when clinicians choose to give an intervention or drug to patients who are more/less severe and likely to have poor/good outcome, which makes the cause-effect analysis difficult to impossible. On the other hand, if we randomize people to usual care or usual care plus the AI tool, and keep all involved blinded, we can learn with scientific rigor what the impact of the AI tool is since the only factor that differed was the AI (Figure 2.2). With randomization, in a sufficiently large study, all other factors should balance out between the control group and the intervention arm. This not only includes the factors that we know, such as age and gender, but also factors that are unknown and importantly those that are not fully understood.

With the first nonrandomized approach, the difference between the groups could be due to the severity of disease or many other factors that go into the decision. Some claim that you can adjust for those differences statistically. The truth is that you can only adjust for a small proportion of those differences, and you never really know how much. In practice, the variables that are needed for this adjustment (e.g., the clinician's thought process) are rarely recorded in the EHR and therefore unavailable for this analysis.

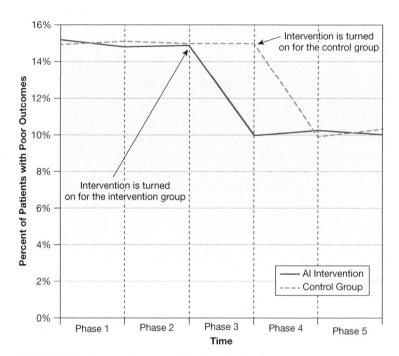

FIGURE 2.2. Graph of a hypothetical randomized controlled trial of AI over time. Randomization provides the machinery to assess if the outcome is improving. During the preimplementation Phases 1 to 2, the intervention group is no different from the control group. During Phase 3, the intervention has improved outcomes for the intervention group compared with the parallel control group. During Phase 4, the randomization is turned off and both groups receive the intervention. By Phase 5, the entire hospital benefits from the new intervention.

Understand what is and what is not in the EHR

When a physician examines a patient to make a diagnosis, only a subset of the findings is available in the EHR. These are the findings that support the diagnosis. AI does not have access to all of the information from the examination.

Statisticians have sometimes overstated how complex statistical methods can resolve problematic studies and data sets. Theoretically, they are correct if the data set contains the necessary covariates, but often a physician will decide on a treatment without recording in the EHR the factors that went into that decision. Even when they are recorded, they are rarely in a structured form that can be used for statistical analyses or AI modeling.

With both approaches above, some patients receive the intervention and some receive usual care. The difference is that with the nonrandom approach the decision is arbitrary (not random but determined by individual preference or convenience) and therefore it is impossible to assess the impact of the intervention on the outcome. This minor difference between arbitrary and random makes a major difference between learning how to improve patient outcomes and not learning. For many interventions, there is clinical equipoise, and the choice of A vs B is often arbitrary. Clinical equipoise is defined as a genuine uncertainty in the expert medical community over whether an intervention or treatment will be beneficial. The change from arbitrary to random is very small but it changes the environment from a nonlearning system to a learning system. With new AI tools, there is almost always clinical equipoise—the experts are uncertain whether this technology will improve patient health without causing unintended consequences compared with usual care.

PRINCIPLE 14 • Recognize an <u>inappropriate control group</u> and a weak study design.

Often people promoting AI products will resist a rigorous randomized study design and propose a much weaker alternative—but impressive sounding. Understanding what is wrong with these weaker study design alternatives is an important modern skill.

Suppose a new AI tool is implemented to identify patients who need early discharge planning preparations because the hospital identified this process as a contributor to prolongation of hospital stays. As part of this program, the hospital hires a transitions care coordinator to improve the planning and handoff process. This person works Monday through Friday and uses the AI tool to risk stratify and identify patients on admission who will need assistance. Rather than randomizing at a patient level (as each is admitted), the hospital administrator plans to use the patients admitted on the weekend as the control group.

Although this may seem reasonable, the evaluation would be completely flawed and would fail to measure the impact of the intervention on the outcome. Choosing just the patients admitted on the weekend to be the control group is not random. They may differ from the patients admitted during the work week in countless ways. Adjusting for these differences statistically is not scientifically possible and therefore does not solve the problem.

> *"Improving study design and minimizing bias are much more important than using complex statistical methods to correct for problems."*
> —JOHN C. BAILAR, III.

When people fail to test AI, they unknowingly, or knowingly, try to persuade others with the weak evaluations (Table 2.3). These methods have their

TABLE 2.3	Study Designs for AI in Health Care That Are Weak Alternatives to a Patient-Level Pragmatic Randomized Controlled Trial

Observational studies with statistical adjustments of confounders
Before-after designs, pre-post comparisons, historical control groups
Quasi-experimental designs
Time series/interrupted time series
Natural experiments
Difference in differences
Propensity score adjustments
Stepped wedge designs
Case-control
Mixed-methods research
Nested case-control
Sequential Multiple Assignment Randomized Trials
Pseudo-randomized controlled trial
Selecting patients who receive an intervention and comparing the results to all other patients
Before-and-after quasi-experimental study with interrupted time series analysis

place, but for testing AI in medicine, these are generally poor options, especially if it is possible to randomize at a patient level—whereby each patient is individually randomized to a group as opposed to randomizing in clusters or groups. Pragmatic trials are those that are conducted within routine clinical care, as opposed to a controlled research environment. Analyzing randomized trials is straightforward since the only difference between the study arms is the intervention. In contrast, complex statistical methods can be used in an attempt to cure the problems with weak studies, but these are band-aids, which rarely solve the underlying problem. Weak study designs often provide the wrong conclusion for AI in health care. Statistically controlling for confounding factors will often make the answer a little bit less wrong—but still wrong.

 "What you said was so confused that one could not tell whether it was nonsense or not."

—WOLFGANG PAULI, THEORETICAL PHYSICIST, NOBEL LAUREATE, 1945.

PRINCIPLE 15 • Create a positive value proposition for the front-line people implementing AI in their workflow. Show them that the personal benefits outweigh the costs.

Clinicians are dedicated to do what is best for their patients, and when they see proof that a new AI approach will help them deliver this, they will be supportive. Answer the question "What's in it for me?" Hospital leaders, administrators, and operations people may not understand why randomization of AI is in their best interest. If we do not help them understand this, they could inadvertently sabotage projects. Randomization of AI tools cannot be forced upon the groups who will implement the tool. They must lead the project.

Rigorous evidence from an RCT will support the long-term funding of internal programs for hospital managers and is therefore in their best interest. Without it, support will fade and there will be yet a different approach each year. So, to be successful, a health care system must retain and promote those who conduct rigorous evaluations because in academic science and medicine this trusted approach applies to the implementation of AI as it does for any new procedure.

Table 2.1 presented flawed AI claims. In contrast to these types of flawed claims, what is needed is a statement like this: "In a recent randomized controlled trial published in [a high-impact journal], patients randomized to the AI arm had significantly improved health outcomes compared with the usual care arm." The remaining chapters of this book teach how to achieve this level of rigor required from a high-profile journal and experience this watershed moment moving from claim to proof and from overstatement to evidence.

PRINCIPLE 16 • Reject the flawed thinking that science slows AI advancement.

Knowledge never slows real progress. AI salespeople have said "We cannot spend 5 years performing a randomized controlled trial to test if our AI product works. We need to use this now." The truth is that randomizing speeds progress. By using a pragmatic randomized trial in a learning health care system framework, many AI systems can be assessed at very low cost.

AI proponents will sometimes reject the use of an RCT stating that an RCT of AI would take 4 to 5 years, which they explain is too long to wait.[3] Some suggest that AI can instead compare patients who were given drug A and those given drug B and use this information to prospectively help doctors prescribe the right drug to patients the first time without trial and error. Although this sounds like an excellent idea, the reality is a bit more nuanced and AI cannot do this in a valid way, due to confounding by indication. This is the type of overpromise that slows widespread implementation. The solution is to find areas of health care that have a specific problem, which a specific AI tool can solve, and avoid pretending that AI is magical and can solve problems that it cannot. Furthermore, many AI tools can be rigorously studied at one hospital in less than 1 year by implementing pragmatic patient-level randomized trials.

Companies that are successful with AI, like Google, Amazon, and Facebook, conduct hundreds of concurrent randomized experiments every day. They do these experiments embedded in their routine work environment. They have adopted this behind-the-scenes randomization approach in a way that customers do not even notice. These are often performed as A/B testing rather than before-after studies. The reason is that the A/B testing is based on randomization and is far superior to before-after studies. Health care organizations often talk for months or years about conducting one experiment of AI. In the future, the successful organizations will conduct many trials of AI every day in adaptive platform frameworks. These trials can study multiple AI implementations and important related questions in a perpetual manner of "keep the winner and drop the loser." Successful health care organization will embrace the culture of "test everything" with randomization as the "secret sauce." Of course, all of this must be performed in an ethical manner with the Institutional Review Board approval.

PRINCIPLE 17 • Medical leaders must educate others to change the culture for the age of AI implementation.

A health care culture that consistently favors action over evidence will not survive. Within a health care system, there can be particularly strong resistance to randomizing AI tools around outcomes that are quality metrics or linked to financial penalties, such as 30-day hospital readmissions. The thinking of some hospital leaders and administrators is often that this end point is so important that we need to assume this new AI tool will result in improvements and bypass the evaluation.

Hospital leaders can improve the culture by changing the goals they assign to their managers and administrators. For example, telling them that you want an action plan implemented to fix hospital readmissions in 60 days is unrealistic and counterproductive. Telling them to reduce readmissions by 3 percentage points next year creates problems. Instead say that you expect them to work with an interdisciplinary team to design a pragmatic RCT to assess whether an AI readmission predictive modeling tool, coupled with an implementation plan, will reduce hospital readmissions in the next year.

Successful hospital leaders will send the right message about rigorous AI evaluations to their managers.

PRINCIPLE 18 • Describe the logic of randomization to others.

Table 2.4 highlights the logic of the RCT.

"I am extraordinarily patient, provided I get my own way in the end."
—Margaret Thatcher.

TABLE 2.4	Randomizing Patients to Usual Care vs Usual Care Plus an AI Model

1. Define usual care for a group of patients.
2. Randomize the patients into two groups but ensure that both groups continue to receive usual care.
3. For one group (a random half), use the AI model to compute the probability of a complication [or another outcome].
4. For those identified to have the highest risk in the random half, triple check that they receive the appropriate prevention measures, which is usual care.
5. Every patient will continue to receive usual care. Nothing will be taken away from any patient.
6. Assess the impact.
7. If effective, apply the AI tool to all patients.

PRINCIPLE 19 • Regression to the mean (RTM) is the Achilles' heel of AI research. Learn to recognize it and avoid flawed conclusions by using stronger study designs.

RTM is one of the most important concepts to understand to truly assess whether AI is having an impact. Surprisingly, few people involved in health care or AI understand RTM even though it was first described by Sir Francis Galton in 1877! This lack of understanding has slowed progress in health care and increased costs.

RTM occurs when one selects outliers at baseline and then assesses these outliers in the future. These outliers nearly always move closer to the mean, or average, of the entire group, without imposing any intervention on them.

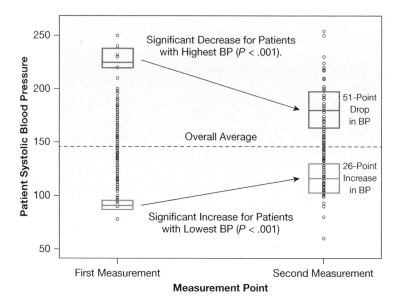

FIGURE 2.3. Regression to the mean. This graph illustrates the statistical phenomenon of regression to the mean in which extremely high or low values will move closer to the average on a second reading. This effect will happen without any intervention. Note that these changes are both statistically and clinically significant. *P* values are based on the Wilcoxon signed-rank test. BP, blood pressure. (Reproduced from Byrne D. *Publishing Your Medical Research*. Wolters Kluwer; 2017. https://www.slideshare.net/DanielByrne12/publishing-your-medical-research-125452257.)

By nature, the outlier will regress to (move close to) the natural mean without any help (Figure 2.3). The problem is that in health care an intervention is often applied to these outliers and the change observed is then taken as evidence that the intervention worked. For example, the group under study is chosen to be the unit in the hospital with the highest rate of infections, or the most patient falls, or the greatest number of readmissions. Or the outlier month in which patient complications are exceptionally high is selected as the starting point for a before and after intervention. This is a flawed design.

"Regression to the mean (RTM) is a statistical phenomenon that can make natural variation in repeated data look like real change. It happens when unusually large or small measurements tend to be followed by measurements that are closer to the mean."

—Adrian Barnett et al[4]

A recent study published in *The New England Journal of Medicine* illustrates this point.[5] The "Hotspotting" program was created to improve outcomes among "Superutilizers," that is patients with very high use of health care services. When the program was later tested in an RCT, it failed, as the authors explain here:

> *"In this randomized, controlled trial involving patients with very high use of health care services, readmission rates were not lower among patients randomly assigned to the Coalition's [hotspotting] program than among those who received usual care."*[5]

If this study had not been randomized, RTM could have been used to misinterpret the findings. It could have been concluded that the hotspotting program did work. The reason is that the patients selected for this program had exceptionally high cost of care before the program and, on average, they moved closer to the mean without any intervention. The authors did a great service by conducting a rigorous randomized control trial, thus showing that the intervention did not work—and also showing that if the study was not randomized it would have provided the wrong answer.

> *"In contrast, a comparison of the intervention-group admissions during the 6 months before and after enrollment misleadingly suggested a 38-percentage-point decline in admissions related to the intervention because the comparison did not account for the similar decline in the control group."*[5]

This type of intervention is also an example of our current reactive health care system's reliance on lagging indicators in a failed way. In the future, successful health care systems will use AI predictive models to create leading indicators (future high utilizers). Lagging indicators are backward-looking metrics, while leading indicators are forward-looking metrics. Before there were accurate and precise AI predictive models, health care was limited to use weak lagging indicators but now AI provides a wealth of valuable leading indicators.

The old mentality of hospital leaders was "If you have a problem in the hospital and you try something, and the results look better, then that is good enough evidence for me." That is the precise definition of RTM. The new mentality is "If a high-profile medical journal would not publish your evaluation, then it is not good enough for me either." Even if you do not plan to publish a paper, there is no reason that you cannot get the right answer and have the same level of rigor in your evaluation of AI.

In studies that have a negative result, researchers sometimes try to use RTM to "prove" that the intervention worked in a subgroup. Surprisingly, this statistical sleight of hand eludes many medical journal reviewers and editors in this form: "Although our intervention did not improve outcomes in the overall study, in a *post hoc* analysis we assessed whether the participants with high baseline levels of X would benefit from this intervention. We found a significant improvement in these high-risk patients." Note: this flawed approach can also be used to show that patients with the low baseline levels of X are made worse by the same intervention! Some will argue that they prespecified the analysis of a subgroup but that does not fix the problem that the conclusion will always be the same based on RTM. If you prespecify that you will look at the patients who had a high baseline level of X, it just means that you planned on using RTM as your "proof." One of the reasons that journals do not catch these statistical flaws is that 58% of medical journal reviewers reported that they lack the statistical skills needed to review the papers they are asked to review.[6]

 FOR MORE INFORMATION

Fundamentals of Clinical Trials. Friedman et al[7]
The Encyclopedia of Biostatistics. Armitage et al[8]

CHAPTER SUMMARY

Science is not the enemy of AI; it is the solution, which will assist health care professionals in continuously learning how to use AI safely and effectively. AI models and AI alerts could actually worsen outcomes, and therefore, the ethical justification for randomization is compelling. Big tech companies run many randomized trials continuously to assess engagement with their online products and health care can learn from their example. A pragmatic RCT of AI in medicine does not need to be difficult, take years to conduct, or disrupt clinical workflows.[9-11] These trials can be frictionless, fast, and low cost. Randomization is the solution—not the problem. Randomization solves many problems that most people are not even aware of.

REFERENCES

1. Wong A, Otles E, Donnelly JP, et al. External validation of a widely implemented proprietary sepsis prediction model in hospitalized patients. *JAMA Intern Med.* 2021;181(8):1065-1070. Erratum in: *JAMA Intern Med.* 2021;181(8):1144.
2. Kelly CJ, Karthikesalingam A, Suleyman M, et al. Key challenges for delivering clinical impact with artificial intelligence. *BMC Med.* 2019;17:195.

3. Chettipally UK. *Punish the Machine!: The Promise of Artificial Intelligence in Health Care.* Advantage Media Group; 2019.

4. Barnett AG, van der Pols JC, Dobson AJ. Regression to the mean: what it is and how to deal with it. *Int J Epidemiol.* 2005;34(1):215-220. Erratum in: *Int J Epidemiol.* 2015;44(5):1748.

5. Finkelstein A, Zhou A, Taubman S, Doyle J. Health care hotspotting—a randomized, controlled trial. *N Engl J Med.* 2020;382(2):152-162.

6. Byrne D. *Publishing Your Medical Research.* Wolters Kluwer; 2017. https://www.slideshare.net/DanielByrne12/publishing-your-medical-research-125452257.

7. Friedman LM, Furberg CD, DeMets DL, Reboussin DM, Granger CB. *Fundamentals of Clinical Trials.* Springer; 2015.

8. Armitage P, Colton T. *Encyclopedia of Biostatistics.* Wiley; 2005.

9. Walker SC, Creech CB, Domenico HJ, French B, Byrne DW, Wheeler AP. A real-time risk-prediction model for pediatric venous thromboembolic events. *Pediatrics.* 2021;147(6):e2020042325.

10. Van Driest SL, Wang L, McLemore MF, et al. Acute kidney injury risk-based screening in pediatric inpatients: a pragmatic randomized trial. *Pediatr Res.* 2020;87(1):118-124.

11. Bloom SL, Stollings JL, Kirkpatrick O, et al. Randomized clinical trial of an ICU recovery pilot program for survivors of critical illness. *Crit Care Med.* 2019;47(10):1337-1345.

3

Evaluation—
The Facts Matter.
Pseudo-Innovation vs
Real Innovation

PRINCIPLE 20 • Learn to speak AI. Familiarize yourself with modern AI terminology.

> *"Though machine learning and big data may seem mysterious at first, they are in fact deeply related to traditional statistical models that are recognizable to most clinicians."*
>
> —ANDREW BEAM AND ISAAC KOHANE.[1]

The world of Artificial Intelligence (AI) has its own terminology and jargon; here is a compilation of the most useful (Table 3.1). This is not meant as a complete dictionary definition of these terms. This is designed to help those in health care understand some of the machine learning (ML) terminology.

Be aware of the "Rashomon effect" with AI claims in medicine

The Rashomon effect is named after the 1950 film, Rashomon, in which four witnesses have very different accounts of a murder. The Rashomon principle, or effect, describes a phenomenon in which individuals seeing the same occurrence, or event, describe the event in different, and often contradictory, ways. This is often seen in health care AI projects due to different backgrounds and training, subjective interpretation, self-interested advocacy, career incentives, or conflicts of interest—rather than an objective truth. Take, for example, how a large multidisciplinary team addresses how to improve hospital readmissions. It is like herding cats. As a result of the Rashomon effect, for thousands of years, medicine made very little impact on the health of patients. By applying appropriate statistical analyses and randomization, however, most observers should arrive at the same conclusion.

TABLE 3.1	AI Terminology Defined for Those in Health Care

AI Terminology	Definition
Recall	Sensitivity, or true positive rate. eg: Among the patients with cancer, what percent did the model predict had cancer?
Precision	Positive predictive value. eg: Among the patients predicted to have cancer, what percent actually had cancer?
Ground Truth	Gold standard.
Class Imbalance	Low event rate or a rare condition, eg, 1% vs 99%.
Imbalanced Data Set	A data set that deviates from 50% with and without the outcome.
Brittleness	Lack of model robustness/stability causing a failure to generalize.
Supervised Learning	A typical predictive model in which patients are labeled as, eg, cancer or benign. A radiologist might label each mammogram and then a model is created to use the features of the image to correctly predict.
Unsupervised Learning	A clustering technique in which patients are not labeled but machine learning methods are used to identify subtypes of a disease.
Feature	Predictor, input, raw, or derived data, eg, an area of an image or a patient characteristic, such as age.
Feature Selection/ Extraction	Variable selection, such as finding a subset of potential predictors needed to create a predictive model.
Manual Feature Engineering/ Construction	A process by which humans derive and select predictors.
Label	Outcome variable that a model is attempting to predict or classify, eg, cancer vs benign.

TABLE 3.1 *Continued*

AI Terminology	Definition
Label/Data Leakage	Reverse causation, eg, long hospital length of stay is not a predictor of a complication but is caused by it; using this as a predictor would artificially improve the performance of the model.
Confusion Matrix	Contingency table.
F_1	Overall measure of a model's accuracy based on the harmonic mean of precision and recall.[2]
Distributional Shift	Changes in data set over time, or from training to implementation.
Training Data Set	Used for the initial model creation.
Validation Data Set/Development Set	A data set used to fine-tune the hyperparameters of a model and assess and rank various models.
Test Data Set	Data set used to assess the performance of the model.
	Note: in health care, this is called the validation data set.
Test	In AI, "test" is the same as "validate" in the medical world.
Training-Test	Derivation-validation data sets.
Hyperparameter	Tuning methods specified by the analyst used to control the AI learning process to create a more accurate model.
Target	Outcome variable, response variable, dependent variable.
Weights	Coefficients.
Loss	Error signal, residual, difference between the predicted and actual outcomes.
Noise	Measurement error.
One-Hot Encoding	Dummy coding.

(continued)

| TABLE 3.1 | *Continued* |

AI Terminology	Definition
Concept Drift	The statistical properties of the outcome change over time.
Learning	Fitting [a predictive model].
To Learn	To fit [a predictive model].
Learners	Predictive models or machine learning algorithms.
A/B Test	Randomized experiment.
Matthews Correlation Coefficient	Pearson's phi coefficient, Yule coefficient.
Greenfield Deployment	Installation of an AI system where previously there was none.
Brownfield Deployment	Upgrade to an existing AI system.
Transfer Learning	The ability to take information gained from solving one AI problem to another situation.

"Everyone is entitled to his own opinion, but not his own facts."

—Senator Daniel Patrick Moynihan.

PRINCIPLE 22 • **From Day 1 of your project, create an unbiased way to assess the internal and external validity and the replication of your AI tool. The best place to start is by studying the 73-page TRIPOD guidelines.**

"A systematic review comparing clinical prediction models based on regression with those based on machine learning revealed troubling weaknesses in model evaluation."

—Michael Pencina et al[3,4]

The following are a few definitions before discussing the mechanics of evaluation: *Internal validation* refers to an evaluation of the performance of a predictive model with the same training data set that was used to develop the model. *External validation* refers to an evaluation of the model with a separate data set. The external validation data set does not need to be from another institution.[5] A *temporal external validation* refers to an evaluation using a separate data set which is collected during a period after the internal validation's data set. A *geographical validation* refers to an evaluation at a different site (at another hospital or a different country). A *split-sample validation* refers to an evaluation in which the training data set is randomly split and then a percentage of it, perhaps 80%, is used for creating the model and 20% is used for the validation.

These external validation analyses will identify models that are flawed due to data dredging, fishing expeditions, falsely claiming benefit in a subgroup, cherry-picking results, or general overfitting. The AI field is mired in a replication crisis and needs more modern validation research to assess the reproducibility of the results from AI models in an unbiased manner. The solution to this crisis is to document rigorous validation and reproducible research in peer-reviewed journals.

This research should be published with complete transparency, including code and data sharing. In the past, models were published but lacked the inclusion of information needed for replication. A statement such as the following can be added to the methods of a paper: "All source code for this work are available at http://github.com...." For an example of proper data and code sharing, see the AlphaFold paper.[6] Data sharing remains a challenge, but the field needs to continue to share more data and coding. Rather than claiming that you cannot share anything, consider attempting to share something, for example, the model's formula, and gradually become more comfortable with this.

The studies must be large enough that the conclusions are valid and rigorous enough that a high-profile medical journal would publish. Do not overmine your data in a reckless way. This means studying an inordinate number of potential predictors yet failing to assess them in a validation study. Instead, raise the level of sophistication to create reproducible research. Do this by prespecifying your external validation in the analysis plan and include the validation in your initial publication.[7] Do not suggest that sometime in the future you, or others, might get around to an external validation. The TRIPOD guidelines are long (73 pages) and detailed but contain a wealth of information. They do not dictate how to build your model, but they do recommend how to report it.

"Delivering the potential of artificial intelligence in clinical decision-making will require testing interventions in well-designed randomized clinical trials and reporting these results in a standardized and transparent fashion."

—NATURE MEDICINE EDITORIAL BOARD.[8]

PRINCIPLE 23 • Convincing clinician colleagues that your model is well validated is as important as convincing biostatisticians.

Although some statisticians prefer to use the full data set to build the model and then use a bootstrap to evaluate it, clinicians are much more impressed by seeing how the models hold up in a new external validation data set. Since clinicians make up the majority of National Institutes of Health study sections and peer reviewers for journals, it is just as important to convince them, as statisticians.

A bootstrap validation is a computer simulation used to see if the model is stable. Is the model overfitting the data to noise? Is it modeling something that happened once that will not be useful in the future uses of this model? For example, a disaster scenario, a change in electronic health record (EHR) vendors, a change in imaging equipment, or a pandemic. How stable is your model? Will it misbehave if put into practice? It is often necessary to have several years of data to predict annual events and account for seasonal effects. Clinicians often favor an external validation over the bootstrap. They are more convinced when they see that the model works in a completely different set of patients. External temporal validations have many advantages over cross-validation methods.[9]

A third alternative (to the bootstrap and external temporal validation) is to randomly split the sample. The advantage of randomly splitting the sample is that if there is a temporal effect across the years that the data was collected the validation will not be impacted. The disadvantage of this approach is that you can be fooled into thinking that the model will predict in the future better than it will. If the sample size is small, the random split may not be the best option.

For many medical AI models, a good solution for most projects is to select the first 80% of the patients from the training data set to build the model. Run a bootstrap validation on this data set. Then perform an external temporal validation on the next 20% of the patients. The bootstrap needs to be used more but not in place of an external temporal validation. Do use the bootstrap more often to provide a 95% confidence interval for variable importance ranks and other important metrics.

Chapter 3 • Evaluation—The Facts Matter. Pseudo-Innovation vs Real Innovation

43

PRINCIPLE 24 • AI must focus on <u>improving hard outcomes</u> that are important to patients—not surrogate end points or process metrics.

"Hard" outcomes are nonsubjective well-defined, patient-important end points with respect to the disease process and reflect how a patient functions, such as one-year survival. "Soft" outcomes require subjective assessment by the researcher or patient, for example, "the patient appears more energetic."

Outcome metrics capture the impact of AI tools on the health status of patients. *Process metrics* are the components of care delivered and capture the work performed or actions implemented, such as the percent of patients with X who are given Y. For example, it is more important to show that a new AI tool reduced the rate of hospital-acquired infections rather than increased compliance with a bundle of care. Examples of process metrics are timeliness of reporting, comprehensiveness of an examination, waiting room time, and percent of patients with asthma who receive an influenza shot. You will want to ensure that your models or those created by vendors focus on outcome metrics that matter to patients and evaluate the validity of the claims made.

About 99% of the population, including educated leaders in health care, can be overly impressed by claims about AI and ML in medicine, which explains the embellishments by some vendors. Here is how to be in the top 1% when evaluating new AI tools:

- Do not accept claims that the model is a black box because it is proprietary. There are many ways to explain how the model works and what the important drivers are—overall and for a given patient.
- Ask AI vendors for a published study from a high-impact peer-reviewed medical journal.
- Only believe results from a randomized controlled trial. Observational studies of AI are problematic.
- Learn how to critically evaluate published medical research findings related to AI and avoid blindly accepting the claims and conclusions. For example, learn how to interpret a calibration plot.
- Do not rely on patient or expert testimonials.
- Ask for a one-year trial period, at no cost, so that you can test it on a random half of your patients.
- Be skeptical of claims that the system is so advanced that it requires new expensive faster computer hardware. AI vendors will sometimes convince hospitals to invest millions of dollars in faster computer hardware because it will be needed for the new AI applications. This is often untrue. Much of the need for expensive hardware is based on faster calculations that are irrelevant in health care. Do not spend millions of dollars on decimal dust.

- Create an AI evaluation committee comprised of members with years of experience in predictive modeling and AI, including a clinical domain expert, an experienced biostatistician, an AI researcher, and a computer scientist.
- Do not accept reports of overall accuracy or high sensitivity without specificity and other metrics—for example, a calibration plot.

PRINCIPLE 25 • Simpler models are often better for low-dimensional, nonimaging, data.

"Entities should not be multiplied beyond necessity."
—Occam's razor or the Law of Parsimony.

Do not attempt to pull the wool over someone's eyes with overly complex AI models and complicated study designs that do not add value. Some AI developers brag about how complex their model is, as if this is a sign of success. But many of these complex models cannot be used in practice—because of their complexity.

"Any intelligent fool can make things bigger and more complex. It takes a touch of genius—and a lot of courage—to move in the opposite direction."
—E. F. Schumacher.

A more parsimonious model which is useful in practice is preferable. The principles of parsimony not only help with transparency but also make the model stable when implemented in the workflow. Those who propose more complex models have the burden of responsibility to demonstrate that the "juice is worth the squeeze." Black box models should not be blindly accepted. How would a more transparent logistic regression (LR) model with fewer predictors perform? Reproducibility and transparency are essential.

"Stop explaining black box machine learning models for high stakes decisions and use interpretable models instead."
—Cynthia Rudin.[10]

If your goal is to use a model in real-time to improve health outcomes, parsimony is not your enemy. Complex models are less likely to be used and accepted.

"Simple models, like logistic regression, often do quite well."
—Professor Peter Szolovits, during his MIT course "Machine Learning for Healthcare".[11]

Some statisticians take pride in making complex models. If the model is so complex that it cannot be implemented, you have accomplished little. After you have about four factors in a model, adding nonlinear terms may not improve the performance of the model. If you increase the complexity of a model, you must demonstrate that the gain in performance outweighs the burden created for the person implementing it.

PRINCIPLE 26 • For many applications in medicine, especially clinical decision support with a binary end point and low-dimensional data, LR is a superior choice over ML.

High-dimensional data sets are those in which there are an overwhelming number of potential predictors (think of pixels in a mammogram), and this number is usually greater than the number of patients in the data set. Examples of high-dimensional data sets include imaging studies (radiology, pathology, dermatology), electrocardiograms, and genetics. Low-dimensional data sets are those in which the number of potential predictors is less than the number of patients and reasonable to evaluate individually. High-dimensional data sets often have complex interaction among the predictors that then require ML approaches.

In the recent medical literature of low-dimensional problems, ML often appeared to be superior, but in many cases, the evaluations were biased. Therefore, higher standards are needed for reporting AI tools. Although there is great excitement about advanced ML, LR often outperforms ML for low-dimensional problems.[4] Many of the overpromises about ML are based on flawed comparisons.[4]

One of the problems with ML is that it will often require a huge number of features/predictors and then becomes difficult to use in practice. ML and other AI tools seem attractive and have often been given somewhat of a free pass in having to demonstrate that they perform appropriately. This needs to change for real progress. An important skill is learning to match the right tool for a particular problem and then being fluent in these various tools to be equally comfortable using them. An agnostic approach to choosing modeling techniques is valuable in creating the best model, publishing in top journals, and obtaining grants.

"We found no evidence of superior performance of ML [machine learning] over LR [logistic regression]. Improvements in methodology and reporting are needed for studies that compare modeling algorithms."

—**Christodoulou et al**[4]

PRINCIPLE 27 • Evaluate the complete set of questions and metrics for a model and do not limit your decision based solely on the AUC.

AUC is the <u>A</u>rea <u>U</u>nder the (receiver-operating-characteristic) <u>C</u>urve, also known as the concordance statistic, concordance index, or c-statistic. This is a measure of the model's discrimination, with 1.0 being perfect and 0.5 being worthless. Discrimination is a metric that answers the question "Do patients with poor outcome have a higher probability from the model than patients with good outcome?" ROC is the Receiver-Operating-Characteristic curve. AUC is the metric. ROC is the graph. The ROC graph plots the sensitivity vs 100-specificity for each predicted probability for a model, that is, 10%, 50%, and 90% (Figure 3.1).

What is a good AUC? This depends, but we know that it typically ranges from 0.5 (worthless) to 1.0 (perfect). The AUC can drop below 0.5; however, this is usually due to an outcome coding error. The comparison being made in the evaluation should be against what the AUC is for the current usual care. If there is currently no risk assessment, then the AUC is ~0.5, so an AUC of 0.65 would be considered an improvement. Many areas of clinical medicine have no risk stratification, or it is performed by humans who are often confident that they can predict it with accuracy. When measured, however, their gestalt AUC is not much better than chance.

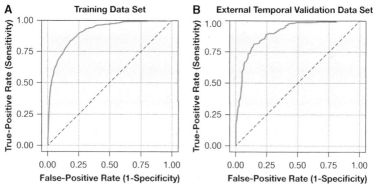

FIGURE 3.1. The receiver-operating-characteristic curve—ROC. Panel A is the ROC curve for the derivation cohort; concordance statistic = 0.908 (95% CI 0.896-0.918). Panel B is the ROC curve for the external temporal validation cohort; concordance statistic = 0.904 (95% CI 0.894-0.913). (Reproduced with permission from Pediatrics, Walker SC, Creech CB, Domenico HJ, French B, Byrne DW, Wheeler AP. A real-time risk-prediction model for pediatric venous thromboembolic events. *Pediatrics.* 2021;147(6):e2020042325. Copyright © 2020, by the, AAP.)

Change the game from "my AUC is better than your AUC" to "this approach improved patient outcomes better than usual care".

> *"When a measure becomes a target, it ceases to be a good measure."*
>
> —GOODHART'S LAW,[12,13]

The ROC, sensitivity, specificity, positive predictive value, and negative predictive value are important but incomplete methods of assessing AI. These *in silico*, computer modeling, evaluations of AI do not provide sufficient evidence. The scientific method of evaluation is the prospective randomized controlled trial in a real-world setting, in which patient outcomes from usual care and the model are compared to outcomes from usual care alone. This evaluation must demonstrate that there was effectiveness without unintended consequences—that the benefits outweigh the risks.

If one only compares the AUC, the conclusion might be that the ML model is superior to the LR model, as in Table 3.2. If, however, one critically examines the two models and answers the remaining dozen questions in Table 3.2, then the LR model is the better option. A common problem is that a group will propose a predictive model that has an AUC that is slightly higher than the comparator and they will conclude that their model is superior. Table 3.3 shows an alternative situation in which deep learning (DL) provides the best option when one evaluates the full list of questions. Logistic regression and ML tools, such as DL, have strengths and weaknesses for different clinical problems. Predicting breast cancer from a mammogram is very different from predicting a pressure injury from a dozen demographic and laboratory values.

> *"...comparisons often fail to take into account important aspects of real problems, so that the apparent superiority of more sophisticated methods may be something of an illusion. In particular, simple methods typically yield performance almost as good as more sophisticated methods, to the extent that the difference in performance may be swamped by other sources of uncertainty that generally are not considered in the classical supervised classification paradigm."*
>
> —DAVID HAND.[14]

Hand DJ. Classifier technology and the illusion of progress. *Stat Sci.* 2006;21(1):1-15. Reprinted with the permission of the Institute of Mathematical Statistics.

TABLE 3.2	Which Model Should We Use to Predict Hospital Complication X?	

	Logistic Regression Model	Machine Learning Model
What is the AUC?	0.81	0.85
Is the model explainable? Is the algorithm transparent?	Yes	No
Can the model be easily coded in the EHR?	Yes	No
Are the predictors available and feasible in practice?	Yes	No
Is the score computed within first 24 hours of admission?	Yes	No
Does the model avoid reverse causation?	Yes	No
Can the model be used at other hospitals or populations?	Yes	No
Has the model been rigorously validated?	Yes	No
Is the AUC uninflated from confounders?	Yes	No
Is there a good calibration in an external data set?	Yes	NA/not shown
Is the model parsimonious?	Yes	No
How many predictors are in the model?	10	47
Is the AUC an improvement over usual care and acceptable?	Yes	Yes

Abbreviations: AUC, area under the receiver-operating-characteristic curve; EHR, electronic health record.

Chapter 3 • Evaluation—The Facts Matter. Pseudo-Innovation vs Real Innovation

49

TABLE 3.3	Which Model Should We Use to Predict Signs of Cancer From a Mammogram?	
	Logistic Regression Model	Deep Learning Model
What is the AUC?	0.55	0.85
Is the model explainable? Is the algorithm transparent?	Yes	Partially
Can the model be easily coded in the EHR?	Yes	Yes
Are the predictors available and feasible in practice?	Yes	Yes
Does the model avoid reverse causation?	No	Yes
Can the model be used at other hospitals or populations?	No	Yes
Has the model been rigorously validated?	No	Yes
Is the AUC uninflated from con-founders?	Yes	Yes
Is there a good calibration?	No	Yes
Is the model parsimonious?	Yes	No
How many predictors are in the model?	10	Many
Is the AUC an improvement over usual care and acceptable?	No	Yes

Abbreviations: AUC, area under the receiver-operating-characteristic curve; EHR, electronic health record.

"When you're fundraising, it's AI. When you're hiring, it's ML. When you're implementing, it's logistic regression."

—DANIELA WITTEN, JUAN M. LAVISTA FERRES, AND OTHERS ON TWITTER.

PRINCIPLE 28 • Deep learning is a tool—not the tool.

A *neural network* (NN), or technically an artificial NN, is an algorithm that is structured in a similar manner to a biological NN. Predictors or features for a NN are inputs. The nodes are then weighted to produce an output. As the model, or algorithm, is fed data, the nodes are weighted to improve the accuracy of the prediction.

DL is an extension of NNs with multiple hidden processing layers. These layers can then discover multiple levels of abstraction. With large data sets, these computational models use backpropagation algorithms to iteratively reweight the layers to discover intricate structures in the data. These methods have led to breakthrough advances that have great potential in medicine. For more information about backpropagation, see Andrew Ng's excellent Coursera lectures. Basically, backpropagation—"backwards propagation of errors"—is an algorithm used in NNs to reduce the prediction errors by iteratively reweighting the predictors and nodes.

Although simpler approaches, such as logistic regression, often perform better overall when designing predictive models based on EHR data,[15] DL has been shown to produce much better results for high-dimensional projects based on imaging analysis, electrocardiograms, speech recognition, drug discovery, genomics, disease phenotyping, protein folding, robotics, and text.

"Deep learning is not magic, it's just a statistical technique with specific strengths and weaknesses."

—GARY MARCUS.

"New methods always look better than old ones. Complicated methods are harder to criticize than simple ones."

—BRAD EFRON.[16]

PRINCIPLE 29 • Ask the right questions when evaluating AI tools (Table 3.4).

Master the skills to evaluate AI model metrics

Understanding how to critically interpret AI model metrics is a modern skill health care leaders must have. The following section includes some basic information you need to get started and focuses on the common type of model that is predicting a binary end point.

TABLE 3.4	Evaluations of AI Tools Should Answer These Questions.[17]

1. <u>Who</u> will the model be used on and when? Is that appropriate given how and when the model was developed? Was the model created from a data set that used variables which were specific to or inclusive of the intended population? What are the unknowns and what assumptions are made?

2. What was the <u>outcome variable</u> and when was it recorded? Is this appropriate given how it will be implemented? What are the assumptions?

3. Will the model need to be <u>updated</u> and if so, how? Is there a plan for regular updating? Are there any issues with this given how the model was created and validated? What are the assumptions?

4. Can the predictors be <u>used at the time</u> they are needed? Was the model created from a data set that used variables that are only available at some latter point in time?

5. Is the model <u>reproducible and transparent?</u> Overly complex "black box" models should not be given a free pass.

6. Has the model been <u>rigorously and transparently validated?</u> Have the discrimination and calibration been adequately evaluated and transparently reported?

7. Has the clinical decision support been <u>run silently</u> for a period to assess the performance? Has it then been tested with randomization?

8. Has the clinical decision support and the implementation been assessed in a randomized controlled trial to ensure that there is <u>more benefit than harm</u>?

PRINCIPLE 30 • Learn how to interpret a confusion matrix.

A confusion matrix, in its simplest form, is a two by two table that is often used to describe the performance of a binary AI classification model (Table 3.5). The confusion matrix can indeed be confusing, but the following information should make it clearer. In the matrix, the number of patients predicted to have a condition is compared with the number of patients who actually have the condition. See Figures 3.2 and 3.3 for

TABLE 3.5 Four Key Elements in the Cells of a Confusion Matrix

Name	Abbreviation	Cell	Definition	Value in Example 1 >1%	Value in Example 2 >2%
True Negative	TN	a	Patients predicted to not have the event, and they do not have the event. This value is high and not used in the precision-recall curve.	100,052	105,031
False Positive "Falsely predicted to be positive"	FP	b	Patients predicted to have the event, but they do not actually have the event.	10,485	5506
False Negative "Falsely predicted to be negative"	FN	c	Patients predicted to not have the event, but they actually do have the event.	247	331
True Positive	TP	d	Patients predicted to have the event and they do have the event.	568	484

	Predicted: NO EVENT	Predicted: YES EVENT	
Actual: NO EVENT	a True Negative= 100,052	b False Positive= 10,485	Number without an Event=110,537
Actual: YES EVENT	c False Negative= 247	d True Positive= 568	Number with an Event=815
	Number predicted to not have an Event=100,299	Number predicted to have an Event=11,053	Grand total=111,352

FIGURE 3.2. Confusion matrix—Example 1, >1%. Using the Children's Likelihood Of Thrombosis example, we can divide patients into those who have a probability of a venous thromboembolism >1% or not and then cross them against the actual results.

	Predicted: NO EVENT	Predicted: YES EVENT	
Actual: NO EVENT	a True Negative= 105,031	b False Positive= 5,506	Number without an Event=110,537
Actual: YES EVENT	c False Negative= 331	d True Positive= 484	Number with an Event=815
	Number predicted to not have an Event=105,362	Number predicted to have a Event=5,990	Grand total=111,352

FIGURE 3.3. Confusion matrix—Example 2, >2%. Using the Children's Likelihood Of Thrombosis example, we can divide patients into those who have a probability of a venous thromboembolism >2% or not and then cross them against the actual results.

example of how the results differ depending on where the predicted probability is set. For example 1, all patients with a risk >1% are considered high risk for this rare complication, and for example 2, all patients with a risk >2% are considered high risk.

To make it less confusing insert the word "predicted" after "false." The false positives are "falsely predicted to be positive." The false negatives are "falsely predicted to be negative."

The confusion matrix is a snapshot of only one point on the ROC. Note that by changing the cut point threshold for the predicted probability, one can improve the sensitivity at the expense of the specificity (Figure 3.4). As you will see in future sections, a more effective way to implement a predictive model is to use the continuous predicted probability and avoid dichotomizing it. Therefore, the metrics in Table 3.6 are not as powerful as the metrics in Table 3.8. Predictive models provide a probability from 0% to 100% for an outcome. It is wise in most cases to use this full spectrum and avoid dividing the patients into low and high risk, for example <90% vs ≥90%.

PRINCIPLE 31 • Understand the bias-variance trade-off.

Bias here refers to an error of <u>underfitting</u> a problem with an overly simplistic predictive model. For example, assuming that a straight line would accurately predict a problem that is clearly nonlinear. Variance is the other extreme—<u>overfitting</u> a problem with an overly complex, nonlinear predictive model (Figure 3.5). Variance is an error of assuming that small noise fluctuations are important. So, there is a trade-off to find the right balance so that the model will work well for future data sets meaning that it will generalize beyond the training data set.

Overfitting, high variance, describes the statistical phenomenon in which a model fits the training data closer than appropriate rather than describing the reality of the clinical relationship. An overfit model appears to have good performance, but it is customized to the training data set too closely and will not perform as well in the future on other data sets—the external temporal validation set. Since the external temporal data set was not used in creating the model, it provides a rigorous standard for evaluation of a model. Properly balancing the bias-variance trade-off means fitting the training data appropriately to improve the accuracy of future predictions. Overall, bias is more important than variance in prediction. When the data set gets large and the number of predictors becomes large, variance handles itself.

Methods of graphing AI model performance

1. Area under the receiver-operating-characteristic curve (AUC/ROC)
2. Calibration curves/plots
3. Precision-Recall Curves/plots (PRCs)

PRINCIPLE 32 • Learn how to create and interpret ROC curves.

The ROC (receiver-operating-characteristic) curve summarizes the trade-off between the sensitivity (true positive rate) and 1-specificity (false positive

case	age	sex	Other predictors	outcome	outcome_probability	threshold=>0.20	threshold=>.50	threshold=>0.60	threshold=>0.90
1	45	0	x, y, z	0	0.1				
2	34	1		1	0.2				
3	12	1		0	0.3				
4	67	0		0	0.4				
5	55	1		0	0.5				
6	71	0		1	0.6				
7	45	0		1	0.7				
8	66	1		1	0.8				
9	67	1		0	0.9				
10	58	0		1	1				
					Sensitivity/Recall	1.00	0.80	0.80	0.20
					Specificity	0.10	0.60	0.80	0.80
					100-Specificity	0.90	0.40	0.20	0.20

FIGURE 3.4. Continuous probabilities of predictors and thresholds. This hypothetical example demonstrates how sensitivity, specificity, and 100-specificity can be computed for various thresholds. Then sensitivity and 100-specificity can be plotted on the ROC curve.

| TABLE 3.6 | Metrics of Classifier Performance for Assessing a Predictive Model With a Binary End Point. These Are Based on Dichotomizing the Predicted Probability for a Confusion Matrix | | | |

Name	Definition/Question	Formula	Cells	Value in Example 1 >1% threshold	Value in Example 2 > 2% threshold
Prevalence	What percent of patients have the event?	Event/Total	$(c + d)/(a+b+c+d)$	$(815/111,352) \times 100 = 0.7\%$	$(815/111,352) \times 100 = 0.7\%$
Sensitivity/ Recall/ Detection Rate (True Positive Rate)	Of those with the event, what percent are predicted to have it? How many of the positive cases were detected?	$TPR = TP/((TP + FN))$	$d/(c + d)$	$(568/815) \times 100 = 69.7\%$	$(484/815) \times 100 = 59.4\%$
Specificity (True Negative Rate)	Of those without the event, what percent are predicted to not have it?	$TNR = SPC = TN/((TN + FP))$ 1-FPR	$a/(a+b)$	$(100,052/(100,052 + 10,485) \times 100 = 90.5\%$	$(105,031/(105,052 + 5506) \times 100 = 95\%$

Precision/ Positive Predictive Value	Of those predicted to have the event, what percent are correct?	PPV = TP/ ((TP + FP) or the predicted yes)	d/(b + d)	(568/11,053) × 100 = 5.1%	(484/5990) × 100 = 8.1%
Negative Predictive Value	Of those predicted to not have the event, what percent are correct?	NPV = TN/ (TN + FN)	a/(a+c)	(100,052/ 100,299) × 100 = 99.8%	(105,031/ 105,362) × 100 = 99.7%
False Positive Rate	Of those without the event, what percent of the time is it predicted yes? How many times do you cry wolf? (This is important with alert alarm fatigue.)	FPR = FP/ (FP + TN)	b/(a+b)	(10,485/10,485 + 100,052) × 100 = 9.5%	(5506/5,506 + 105,031) × 100 = 5.0%
False Discovery Rate	Of those predicted yes, what percent do not have the event?	FDR = FP/ (FP + TP)	b/(b + d)	(10,485/ (10,485 + 568)) × 100 = 94.9%	(5,506/(5,506 + 484)) × 100 = 91.9%

(continued)

TABLE 3.6 *Continued*

Name	Definition/Question	Formula	Cells	Value in Example 1 >1% threshold	Value in Example 2 > 2% threshold
False Negative Rate	Of those with the condition, what percent are not correctly predicted?	$FNR = FN/(FN + TP)$	$c/(a+c)$	$(247/(247 + 568)) \times 100 = 30.3\%$	$(331/(331 + 484)) \times 100 = 40.6\%$
Overall Accuracy	Overall, how often is the model correct?	$ACC = (TP + TN)/(total) = Correct/All$	$(a+d)/(a+b+c+d)$	$((568 + 100,052)/111,352) \times 100 = 90.4\%$.	$((484 + 105,031)/111,352) \times 100 = 94.8\%$
Balanced Accuracy	What is the average of sensitivity and specificity?	$BA = (Sensitivity + Specificity)/2$	$((d/(c+d)) + (a/(a+b)))/2$	80.1%	77.2%

Matthews Correlation Coefficient	What is the correlation between predicted and actual cells in the confusion matrix? Also referred to as the phi coefficient or the Yule phi coefficient	MCC = TP*TN − FP*FN/sqrt((TP + FP)*(TP + FN)*(TN + FP)*(TN + FN))	d*a − b*c/ sqrt((d + b)*(d + c)*(a + b)*(a+ c))	0.172	0.206
No Information Rate	What would the accuracy be if there was no information? Used as a bar to evaluate whether human evaluators and various AI methods exceed it.	NIR=Larger outcome group/total	(a+b)/(a+b + c + d)	110.537/ 111,352 × 100 = 99.3%	110.537/ 111,352 × 100 = 99.3%

110,537/ 111,352 × 100 = 99.3%

(continued)

TABLE 3.6 *Continued*

Name	Definition/Question	Formula	Cells	Value in Example 1 >1% threshold	Value in Example 2 > 2% threshold
Misclassification Rate or Error Rate	Overall, how often the model is wrong?	1—accuracy. (FP + FN)/ total = Incorrect/All	(b + c)/ (a+b + c + c)	((10,485 + 247)/ 111,352) × 100 = 9.6%	((5506 + 331)/ 111,352) × 100 = 5.2%
Null Error Rate	How often you would be wrong is you always predicted the larger group?	If majority are yes = Actual no/ Total If majority are no = Actual yes/ Total	(c + d)/ (a+b + c + d)	815/111,352 × 100 = 0.7% (same as the prevalence in this case)	815/111,352 × 100 = 0.7% (same as the prevalence in this case)

F_1-Score	What is the weighted average of the true positive rate (recall) and precision?	$2 \times$ (Precision $\times$ Recall)/(Precision + Recall) $F_1 = 2 \times$ TP/(2 $\times$ TP + FP + FN)	$(2 \times d)/(2 \times (d + b + c)$	$(2 \times 568)/((2 \times (568 + 10,485 + 247) = 0.096$ $(1136)/(11868) = 0.096$ (9.6%) An F_1-Score is a measure of a model's accuracy and is based on the precision and recall.	$(2 \times 484)/((2 \times (484 + 5506 + 331) = (968)/(12,642) = 0.077 \ (7.7\%)$ An F_1-Score is a measure of a model's accuracy and is based on the precision and recall.
Detection Prevalence	What is the number of predicted positive events (both true positive and false positive) divided by the total number of predictions?	Predicted/ Total positive class predictions made as a proportion of all predictions	$(b + d)/(a+b + c + d)$	$(11,053/ 111,352) \times 100 = 9.9\%$	$(5,990/ 111,352) \times 100 = 5.4\%$

(continued)

TABLE 3.6 *Continued*

Name	Definition/Question	Formula	Cells	Value in Example 1 >1% threshold	Value in Example 2 > 2% threshold
Bookmaker Informedness	How similar is the model to random guessing?	BM=(sensitivity + specificity) −100.	(d/(c + d) +a/(a+ b))−100	(69.7% + 90.5%) −100% = 60.2%	(59.4% + 95.0%) −100% = 54.4%
Markedness	What is the probability that prediction is marked vs chance?	MK = PPV + NPV − 1	d/(b + d) +a/ (a+c) −100%	(5.1% + 99.8%) −100% = 4.9%	(8.1% + 99.7%) −100% = 7.8%
	A measure of trust-worthiness of positive and negative predictions by the model.				

TABLE 3.7	Which Predictive Model Is Best for Identifying Patients With Undiagnosed Hemochromatosis?		
	Model 1	**Model 2**	**Model 3**
Accuracy	99.6%	83%	0.4%
Probability of Hemochromatosis =	0 (the model predicts no one has hemochromatosis)	A continuous probability from a logistic regression model, such as: $1/(1 + e^{-z})$ $Z = -15.4 + RDW \times 0.179 + Age \times -0.023....$	1 (the model predicts everyone has hemochromatosis)
AUC	0.5	0.86	0.5

Note: The prevalence of hemochromatosis = 0.4%.

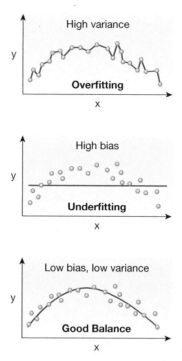

FIGURE 3.5. Bias-variance trade-off. The goal of an AI predictive model is to have both low bias and low variance. Models that are underfit, such as a straight line, have high bias and low variance. Models that are overfit to the training data have low bias and high variance and will not perform well in external temporal validation studies. (Adapted from https://towardsdata-science.com/understanding-the-bias-variance-tradeoff-165e6942b229.)

rate) for a predictive model using the many different probability thresholds.[17,18] Pseudo-innovation is easy to spot when someone brags about only their sensitivity but does not also provide the specificity (or other metrics). By selecting an extreme probability threshold, it is always possible to report an excellent sensitivity but by itself this is meaningless.

PRINCIPLE 33 • **Understand how to create and interpret a calibration curve.**

Model calibration describes how well-predicted probabilities from a model corresponded to observed results (Figure 3.6). The graph is created by plotting a smoothed curved line with a nonparametric locally weighted scatterplot

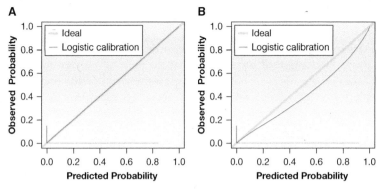

FIGURE 3.6. Calibration curve. Calibration curve for venous thromboembolism risk-prediction Children's Likelihood Of Thrombosis model. In panel A, the derivation cohort calibration curve is illustrated. In panel B, the validation cohort calibration curve is illustrated. (Reproduced with permission from Pediatrics, Walker SC, Creech CB, Domenico HJ, French B, Byrne DW, Wheeler AP. A real-time risk-prediction model for pediatric venous thromboembolic events. *Pediatrics.* 2021;147(6):e2020042325. Copyright © 2020, by the, AAP.)

smoothing plot showing the relationship between predicted values and average of the outcome.[19] Calibration performance is vitally important in AI research and needs to be evaluated, compared, and reported. Calibration also needs to be reported for subgroups (gender, race, etc). Compare the calibration curve with the 45-degree line of identity. Too many AI papers simply report the c-statistics (AUC) but fail to also show the calibration plot. This needs to change. More AI publications need to include a modern calibration curve, which is as important, if not more important than the ROC. Many ML methods will have a slightly better ROC than logistic regression, but the calibration is often much worse (although rarely reported). The calibration from the training data set is not as important as the calibration curve from the external validation data set. We would expect the calibration from the training data set to look impressive. The important test is the calibration plot using new data.

To avoid simplistic binning of the predicted probabilities into deciles, instead use continuous predicted values with a smoother. Calibration curves should be used rather than the outdated Hosmer-Lemeshow statistical test for goodness of fit approach. The problems with the Hosmer-Lemeshow test are it has low power, is hard to interpret, but more important different software will give different results based on where the deciles are arbitrarily drawn producing very different *P* values.

PRINCIPLE 34 • Know how to create and interpret a precision-recall curve (PRC).

Precision is the positive predictive value for the model and recall is the sensitivity. Precision-recall curves summarize the trade-off between these two metrics for a predictive model using the many different probability thresholds (Figure 3.7). The F_1 metric is sometimes used to summarize the PRC as the harmonic mean of precision and recall, but this metric is not ideal.

All three of these performance graphs have strengths and weaknesses with different data sets and clinical problems. They each add value and should all be graphed and displayed for full transparency. In a paper, they can be presented as a figure with multiple panels.

Spectrum bias is a problem that can arise from creating a model based on a data set where 50% of the patients have the outcome and 50% do not. These artificially balanced data set can make it easier to create some AI models but obviously cause problems when the model is deployed in a population that has a different spectrum of patients.

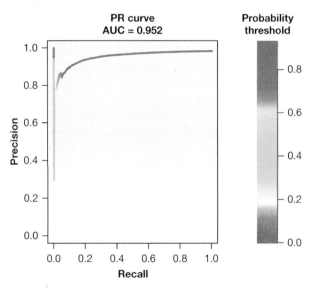

FIGURE 3.7. Precision-recall curve. This graph illustrated the relationship between recall (sensitivity) on the X-axis vs precision (positive predictive value) on the Y-axis for various thresholds from a predictive model. The heatmap on the right illustrates the threshold. Note: true negatives are not used in the precision-recall curve.

PRINCIPLE 35 • Identify an accuracy scam, which is one of the most common forms of pseudo-innovation in hyping AI.

> *It ain't what you don't know that gets you into trouble.*
>
> *It's what you know for sure that just ain't so.*
>
> —MARK TWAIN.

"The AI model has 99% accuracy!" This statement by itself is meaningless but will fool 99% of the population.

AI developers and researchers sometimes mislead people in health care by describing how an AI product has a high overall accuracy. They will claim that they have a predictive model that is 99% accurate, for example. The people making the spending decisions often lack the statistical training to see that this is meaningless. Elizabeth Holmes, the founder of Theranos, bamboozled billions of dollars from investors with misleading claims, such as overall accuracy.[20]

PRINCIPLE 36 • Use the continuous probability when possible and the metrics associated with it.

Most AI models provide a probability from 0% to 100% for prediction of the outcome. This continuous probability contains valuable information and should be used in practice. Many users or developers will chop the predicted probability into two parts, such that less than a 50% probability of a given outcome indicates low risk and great than a 50% probability of a given outcome indicated a high risk. These users will then report the metrics in Table 3.6.

Although occasionally this dichotomization is necessary, many times it is possible to find a way to avoid this dichotomization and, in its place, use the continuous probability from 0% to 100%. The continuous predicted probability is much more powerful and should be used whenever possible (Table 3.8).[21,22]

Overall accuracy (proportion classified correctly), sensitivity (recall), specificity, and precision are all improper accuracy scoring rules, and by themselves, are weak metrics (Figure 3.8). They lack power and can be manipulated to take advantage of unsophisticated consumers. Because these metrics dichotomize the predicted probability and use discontinuous scoring methods, they should be deemphasized. Better metrics are the ROC/AUC, calibration curves, and Brier scores. See Table 3.8. Rather than ask what the sensitivity is, ask what the AUC is, and ask to see the calibration curve. Those who brag about the sensitivity in isolation are probably guilty of pseudo-innovation. Also, ask to see a dot plot of the strength of the predictors (Figure 3.9).

TABLE 3.8 Metrics of Performance for Assessing a Predictive Model With a Binary End Point. These Are Based on Using the Continuous Predicted Probability (as Opposed to the Dichotomized Variable for a Confusion Matrix)

Metric	Definition	Interpretation	Example Value
Discrimination			
AUC (ROC)/c-Statistics/	Area under the receiver-operating-characteristic curve	Measure of the model's discrimination performance 1 = perfect model. 0.5 = worthless model.	0.907
AUPRC	Area under the precision-recall curve	1 = perfect model.	0.952
Brier Score Quadratic Error Measure	Mean squared error of prediction.	When comparing several models, the one with the lower score is superior, but the actual Brier score has limited value. 0 = perfect accuracy, 1 = perfect inaccuracy	0.007
Calibration			
Calibration Slope	A measure of the agreement between the predicted and actual results.	Ideal = 1 Together with the calibration intercept provides a measure of calibration.	0.876
Calibration Intercept	A measure of the actual outcomes at the point where the probability is zero.	Ideal = 0 Together with the calibration slope provides a measure of calibration.	−0.462

	No Hemochromatosis	Hemochromatosis	Total
Predicted No	996	4	1000
Predicted Yes	0	0	0
Total	996	4	1000
Overall accuracy = (996 + 0)/1000 = 99.6%			

FIGURE 3.8. Overall accuracy. This hypothetical example shows why overall accuracy is a weak metric. A model that predicts that no one has hemochromatosis can have an overall accuracy of 99.6% but is completely worthless.

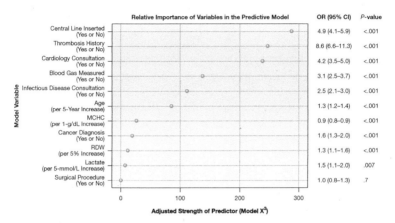

FIGURE 3.9. Dot plot of the strength of predictors. This is a visual representation of the predictors used in the Children's Likelihood Of Thrombosis venous thromboembolism risk-prediction model. Scores are ordered by the adjusted strength of the predictor as quantified by model χ^2 statistic. The table also includes the OR for each variable, along with the 95% CI and P values. (Reproduced with permission from Pediatrics, Walker SC, Creech CB, Domenico HJ, French B, Byrne DW, Wheeler AP. A real-time risk-prediction model for pediatric venous thromboembolic events. *Pediatrics.* 2021;147(6):e2020042325. Copyright © 2020, by the, AAP.)

Here is an example of how some try to show proof when there is little by using overall accuracy. Suppose a model had a poor overall accuracy in a clinic in which 50% of the patients had disease X. To inflate the impression of this model's ability to predict, one would show the model's overall accuracy performance in a population that had a very low rate of disease X. A more accurate and true way to report validity of the model would be to report the metrics in Table 3.8.

For an example of why overall accuracy is the incorrect way to evaluate AI, see Table 3.7.

PRINCIPLE 37 • Learn how to use and interpret the robustness of model metrics (Table 3.8).

> *"Everything should be made as simple as possible, but no simpler."*
> —ALBERT EINSTEIN.

ℹ FOR MORE INFORMATION

Making Sense of the Confusion Matrix. Kevin Markham.[23]
The No Confusion Matrix! Kimberly Fessel.[24]
StatQuest. Josh Starmer.[25]
Statquest—Machine Learning Fundamentals: Bias and Variance. Josh Starmer.[26]
Bias/Variance (C2W1L02). DeepLearningAI. Andrew Ng.[27]
Neural Networks, Deep Learning & AI. Frans Rodenburg.[28]
https://www.youtube.com/watch?v=f0q_sSqNIJc.

CHAPTER SUMMARY

The question is not whether the model is perfect. The question is whether a slightly imperfect model can be used to focus resources and improve health compared with usual care. For many applications of AI in medicine, the optimal implementation is to use the continuous probability of the outcome (0%-100%) rather than the dichotomized version (low risk vs high risk).

Many models can be useful without a high level of precision at the upper tail of the calibration plot. If a hospitalized patient has more than a four-fold increase in the risk of a complication, does it matter if the risk is 91% or 89% if all patients with a risk above 30% receive the prevention? A mindset that an AI project needs to be flawless before it can be deployed leads to project paralysis. Instead view the project as a continuous quality improvement project in an adaptive platform trial. The quality improvement label is sometimes used in health care as an excuse for not randomizing, but true quality improvement is rigorous, includes randomization, and is a necessary component of implementation.

The results should be reported in high-profile medical journals with greater transparency and a detailed appendix—strive for reproducible research using modern robust methods. External validations, with calibration curves, should be included in the initial publication. Journal editors and reviewers can insist on external validations and adherence to modern reporting guidelines. High-quality real-world evidence of AI's true impact in medicine is desperately needed to improve trust and adoption.

REFERENCES

1. Beam AL, Kohane IS. Big data and machine learning in health care. *JAMA*. 2018;319(13):1317-1318.
2. Penha F. Data science bits. The definitive guide to F1 score. Accessed September 19, 2022. https://www.youtube.com/watch?v=_OCYto4zK0g
3. Pencina MJ, Goldstein BA, D'Agostino RB. Prediction models—development, evaluation, and clinical application. *N Engl J Med*. 2020;382(17):1583-1586.
4. Christodoulou E, Ma J, Collins GS, Steyerberg EW, Verbakel JY, Van Calster B. A systematic review shows no performance benefit of machine learning over logistic regression for clinical prediction models. *J Clin Epidemiol*. 2019;110:12-22.
5. Moons KG, Altman DG, Reitsma JB, et al. Transparent reporting of a multivariable prediction model for Individual Prognosis or Diagnosis (TRIPOD): explanation and elaboration. *Ann Intern Med*. 2015;162:W1-W73.
6. Jumper J, Evans R, Pritzel A, et al. Highly accurate protein structure prediction with AlphaFold. *Nature*. 2021;596(7873):583-589.
7. Kahan BC, Forbes G, Cro S. How to design a pre-specified statistical analysis approach to limit p-hacking in clinical trials: the Pre-SPEC framework. *BMC Med*. 2020;18(1):253.
8. Nature Medicine Editorial Board. Setting guidelines to report the use of AI in clinical trials. *Nat Med*. 2020;26(9):1311.
9. Bates S, Hastie T, Tibshirani R. Cross-validation: what does it estimate and how well does it do it? https://arxiv.org/abs/2104.00673
10. Rudin C. Stop explaining black box machine learning models for high stakes decisions and use interpretable models instead. *Nat Mach Intell*. 2019;1:206-215.
11. Szolovits P. MIT course "Machine Learning for Healthcare." https://www.youtube.com/watch?v=wDLzLN1tArA
12. Goodhart C. Goodhart's law. In: Rochon L, Rossi S, eds. *The Encyclopedia of Central Banking*. Edward Elgar Publishing; 2015:227-228.
13. Strathern M. "Improving ratings": audit in the British University system. *Eur Rev*. 1997;5:305-321.
14. Hand DJ. Classifier technology and the illusion of progress. *Stat Sci*. 2006;21(1):1-15.
15. Jung K, Shah NH. Implications of non-stationarity on predictive modeling using EHRs. *J Biomed Inf*. 2015;58:168-174.
16. Efron-B. Comment on statistical modeling: the two cultures. *Stat Sci*. 2001;16(3):218-219.
17. Hand DJ, Till RJ. A simple generalisation of the area under the ROC curve for multiple class classification problems. *Mach Learn*. 2001;45(2):171-186.
18. Byrne D. *Publishing Your Medical Research*. Wolters Kluwer; 2017. https://www.slideshare.net/DanielByrne12/publishing-your-medical-research-125452257
19. Steyerberg EW. *Clinical Prediction Models—A Practical Approach to Development, Validation, and Updating*. Springer; 2019.
20. Carreyrou J. *Bad Blood: Secrets and Lies in a Silicon Valley Startup*. Knopf; 2018.

21. Moons KG, Harrell FE. Sensitivity and specificity should be de-emphasized in diagnostic accuracy studies. *Acad Radiol.* 2003;10(6):670-672.

22. Royston P, Altman DG, Sauerbrei W. Dichotomizing continuous predictors in multiple regression: a bad idea. *Stat Med.* 2006;25(1):127-141.

23. Markham K. Making sense of the confusion matrix. https://www.youtube.com/watch?v=8Oog7TXHvFY

24. Fessel K. The NO CONFUSION matrix! https://www.youtube.com/watch?v=_cpiuMuFj3U

25. Starmer J. StatQuest. https://www.youtube.com/c/joshstarmer

26. Starmer J. StatQuest. Machine learning fundamentals: bias and variance. https://www.youtube.com/watch?v=EuBBz3bI-aA

27. Ng A. Bias/Variance (C2W1L02). DeepLearningAI. https://www.youtube.com/watch?v=SjQyLhQIXSM

28. Rodenburg F. Neural Networks, Deep Learning & AI. https://www.youtube.com/watch?v=f0q_sSqNlJc

Synergy—Building a Successful Clinician-Computer Collaboration

PRINCIPLE 38 • **Successful AI systems provide support and are easy to adopt.**

Everyday Artificial Intelligence (AI) computer systems and human beings enjoy a successful interaction that makes life better. For example, most drivers use a GPS (Global Positioning System) to help them navigate. The GPS provides valuable decision support—but not decision replacement. The GPS did not make the driver obsolete; it added value to the driver. The GPS is generally better at navigating. The human is better at driving. Working together in harmony, each does what it is strong at, and the result is a successful trip to a selected destination. AI saves the driver time, prevents the stress of becoming lost, and enables the driver to focus on driving safely.

For large delivery and transportation organizations such as FedEx, UPS, Uber, and Lyft who are managing many drivers, GPS is an important part of their business strategy. AI provides an optimal route based on updated traffic information and an accurate estimated time of arrival. The drivers can focus on driving safely and will have a better track record for arriving on time. This synergy improves the driver's experience, the delivery organization's profits, and customer's satisfaction. Similarly, AI tools in concert with physicians, and the health care system, should have a positive effect for the patient.

PRINCIPLE 39 • **AI must reduce burden with minimal unintended consequences.**

Let's stay with the GPS example for a moment. Most of us may now notice a decrease in our own navigational and map reading skills as we come to rely on GPS devices. Patients fear this will happen in health care. So, the question is whether or to what extent is this acceptable. What is an acceptable transfer of responsibilities from humans to computers? For clinical care and medical training, this transfer needs to be monitored for skill degradation and automation bias, in which clinicians become complacent and overly reliant on AI.

In Chapter 3, we discussed evaluating AI tools for accuracy and precision. Now we evaluate their impact on the everyday experiences of clinicians and health care providers.[1] For example, clinicians spend an inordinate amount of time on electronic health record (EHR) documentation, wishing they had more time to spend interacting with patients and their families. New AI tools can help solve this problem and add value by prioritizing clinical worklists.

> *"Using high-quality research to carefully validate the most clinically valuable tools for clinical practice will help reduce the burden on physicians and protect subjects."*
>
> —ZHOU ET AL[2]

As you develop a model, assess if it is easily adopted but also for unintended consequence of clinical decision support.[3] A major source of mistrust and outright rejection of AI are the concerns that it will serve to replace the health care provider. But how can this concern be attenuated? Evaluate if implementation of the AI tool causes a decrease in physician skill level.

For some AI applications, the tools may actually improve the level of skill in physicians. If the AI tool provides more time for the physician to spend with patients and less with the EHR, then the evaluation should also assess the impact that has on the patient downstream. A common way to quantify physicians' skills level is with a kappa statistic. This statistical test will measure physician agreement with a gold standard. Other ways to assess skill level are the inter-rater reliability and intra-rater reliability. The main three questions are as follows: (1) How well do physicians agree with the gold standard? (2) How well do physicians agree with one another? and (3) How well do physicians agree with themselves? For more about this, see Lyell et al.[4]

Randomization at the patient level is one of the best solutions for assessing unintended consequences as shown in the following example. A new hospital readmission predictive model was created and displayed in the EHR. After 6 months, several hospital administrators noticed that the hospital length of stay had increased. Initially, it was assumed that the readmission model was to blame, speculating that once the physicians saw a high probability of readmissions in the EHR the physician decided to keep the patient in the hospital longer. Fortunately, the team had randomized the model and was able to show that the length of stay was identical in the two arms. Without randomization, the hospital administrators could have used this concern to turn off the model and halt forward progress of AI in general. Other study designs, such as before-after and those in Table 2.3 would, have no value in solving this problem.

PRINCIPLE 40 • Physicians will embrace AI tools when they see them as a method of intelligence amplification.

In medicine, optimal health care is the result of optimal decision-making. Ideally, we build a work environment which permits computers do what they do best—predict and compute—and affords humans time do what they do best—prevent, diagnose, and treat.

> *"Clinicians should seek a partnership in which the machine predicts (at a demonstrably higher accuracy), and the human explains and decides on action."*
>
> —VERGHESE ET AL[5]

Since much of medicine is decision-making in the face of uncertainty, the combination of clinician and computer decreases the uncertainty and improves the decision-making process. Daniel Kahneman won the Nobel Prize for his brilliant research on this subject.[6] Applying his findings to the implementation of AI in medicine will be a key to success.

Kahneman showed that humans are generally not as skilled at complex statistical computations since this requires weighing an overwhelming number of factors simultaneously. Computers excel at this type of "System 2" thinking, which is deliberative and logical. Humans do well at System 2, but excel at "System 1" thinking, which is fast, intuitive, automatic, and ideal for problem solving. An implementation that combines the best of each system provides an intelligence amplification that results in better decisions. For example, a computer AI model could identify which patient is most likely to have an unexpected death in the hospital. A physician would confirm, assess, and decide on the appropriate treatment.

> *"Combining machine-learning software with the best human clinician "hardware" will permit delivery of care that outperforms what either can do alone."*
>
> —CHEN ET AL[7]

The goal is to have clinicians adopt AI models as their complementary work partners. AI will augment a specific task, not automate an entire job in health care. Success requires leveraging the scalable, fast, and economical benefits of AI to predict and classify many clinical events.

The goal is not to have a self-driving ambulance bring patients to a self-treating hospital.

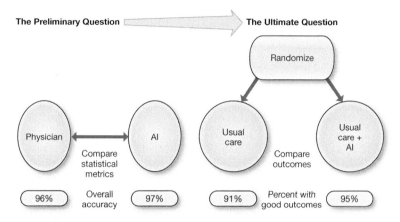

FIGURE 4.1. Randomization of usual care vs usual care plus AI. The preliminary question is whether AI outperforms the physician. The ultimate question is whether AI can improve patient health compared with usual care.

> *"To ask the right question is already half the solution to a problem."*
>
> —CARL JUNG.

The wrong question is whether the AI outperforms the physician. The correct question is whether the combination of a physician with AI clinical decision support results in better patient outcome compared with usual care (Figure 4.1). AI will gradually transform medical decision-making by providing decision support tools that add value and save time.

PRINCIPLE 41 • Be prepared to show clinicians that the AI tool will meet their needs.

To reach a synergistic relationship, AI developers and researchers must study the stumbling blocks and prepare to have compelling and evidence-based answers to the questions in Table 4.1.

Demonstrate that AI converts information overload into one actionable number or alert that provides value and saves time. A nurse, for example, could spend 20 minutes reviewing information about pressure injury (ulcer) risk or instead use the AI-derived probability of pressure injury. In a hospital with 700 patients, this would require 233 hours, or 29 extra nurses (233/8). The hospital computer performs this for free in a split second and then ranks all 700 patients based on risk level. The patients are quickly triaged to speed

TABLE 4.1	Questions That Clinicians May Ask Before Embracing an AI Tool

Why is this needed?

Will this help my patients?

What is the impact on my workflow?

Will this tool be disruptive?

Will there be many false alarms creating alert fatigue?

What is the validity of the model?

What is the value in making this change?

Will this be more efficient than the current workflow?

Will this accurately conduct tedious tasks freeing up value time for my team?

Will this replace me?

decision-making at the point of care. This approach allows nurses to be more productive by focusing on high-risk patients. It provides value and saves time.

The burden of tedious and duplicative tasks contributes to nurse burnout. This problem is so common that there is a recurring journal article titled: "Choosing Wisely: Things We Do For No Reason" in the *Journal of Hospital Medicine*. Nursing burnout, resignations, and job vacancies are major problems, but AI tools can help by removing layers of tedious work. Randomization prevents nurses from becoming burdened with additional AI work—until it is proven to be beneficial. Randomization can also remove layers of work for nurses—if they are proven worthless, such as postdischarge phone calls and daily bathing with chlorhexidine.[8,9]

>*"People should stop training radiologists now. It is just completely obvious that within 5 years deep learning is going to do better than radiologists."*
>
>—GEOFFREY HINTON,[10] 2016.

PRINCIPLE 42 • <u>Show the need</u> for a new AI tool.

Show that a new AI tool is needed by measuring the inability of clinicians to predict an outcome or demonstrate the low clinician inter-rater and intra-rater reliability. Others have shown the need by measuring the wide variability of clinician performance. For example, showing radiologists the wide variability in the sensitivity, specificity, and positive predictive value for

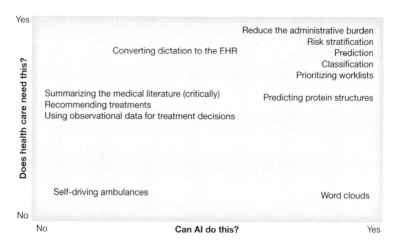

FIGURE 4.2. Graph of what AI can perform vs what health care needs. Success requires focusing on project that is in the upper right corner of this graph. EHR, electronic health record.

a group of radiologists evaluating mammograms for breast cancer can compel them to test the value of a new AI decision support tool that has less variability (Figure 4.2).

Acceptance of AI decision support requires the developers to <u>research and demonstrate why clinicians currently make decision errors</u>. This can be from a variety of reasons including the "availability heuristic" in which clinicians do not have the data they need, causing them to heavily weigh their decision on recent experiences, say a lecture they heard, or article that they read recently. AI can often be more powerful and unbiased in this respect.

Another cause of clinical decision error is "confirmation bias," which is the tendency to find, interpret, and give more weight to information that supports the clinician's diagnosis. For more detail read "*Thinking, Fast and Slow*."[6]

In addition to showing clinicians there is a need for a new AI tool, they must also be convinced that AI algorithms do not function, nor do they strive to function, in the same way that humans think. Daniel and Richard Susskind[11] described the "AI Fallacy" as the mistaken assumption that the only way to develop systems that perform tasks at the level of experts or higher is to replicate the thinking process of human specialists. Just as the first attempts at flying machines were based on the mechanics of birds, the first evolution of AI was rule based and structured like human thinking (if age >65, 2 points; if BMI>30, 1 point, etc.). Then deep learning produced superior results.

PRINCIPLE 43 • Clinicians must be <u>free to overrule</u> any AI recommendation. Algorithms alone should not be making health decisions.

A successful AI system in health care does not take humans out of the process. For example, AI identifies high-risk patients but does not dictate actions to take. The clinical care team reviews the high-risk patients and decides what to do. Here is an example. A predictive model was automated in the EHR identifying patients at high risk for 30-day hospital readmissions. A multidisciplinary team reviewed the patients and found that each of the high-risk patients needed something but there was no one thing they all needed. The most common needs included home health care after discharge, hospice, palliative care, drug rehabilitation, psychiatric consultation, the sickle cell program, and transfer to another hospital, rehabilitation facility, or skilled nursing home. Effective AI identifies the high-risk patients but does not attempt to make decisions about the needed services. Qualified providers handle this as part of a healthy computer-clinician synergy.

As the next step, the developers could suggest various implementation methods for deployment and assess overall outcome impact when combined with the risk model. Here are some readmission examples. The HOMERuN study demonstrated that the patients who were readmitted did not require a new innovative expensive intervention. What they needed was routine care, performed reliably—there was a "know-do" gap.[12] Some interventions that were once thought to reduce readmission, such as a postdischarge phone call, have been shown to have no impact on hospital readmissions.[8] Medication reconciliation programs also had no impact on reducing readmissions.[13] Vanderbilt researchers have demonstrated that the most promising interventions must occur during the hospital stay, not after discharge.[14] Therefore, the probability of hospital readmission needs to be computed on admission and updated daily.

The AI model should also be designed to flag patients when it cannot provide a reliable prediction. Models must notify the clinician with a message such as "The model is unable to provide a reliable prediction for this patient. Please review carefully." Adding 95% confidence intervals (CIs) to a predicted value can also be useful. For example, a 75% risk of an outcome with 95% CI of 73% to 77% will be interpreted differently than a 75% risk of an outcome with a 95% CI of 55% to 95%. Although models should be trained on a diverse population, there will always be patients that are underrepresented, and therefore, it is essential that the model displays the level of uncertainty for these patients.

"Predictions without uncertainty quantification are neither predictions nor actionable."

—EDMON BEGOLI ET AL[15]

PRINCIPLE 44 • Design a <u>frictionless</u> nondisruptive point of care AI user interface. The technology should run silently in the background.

A frictionless system that requires no clinician effort and instead automatically computes a risk probability is more likely to be adopted. An AI system must save time, provide a more precise estimate of risk, and fit seamlessly into the current workflow or ordering system. The process must be easier to "go with the flow" than to find a way to work around it. The user interface must make it easier to do the right thing and harder to do the wrong thing. Aim for a process that does not even ask for one more click. Rather than blame the users for not using an AI tool, work with experts in human factors engineering to study the problem and improve. Study the difference between AI tools that are frictionless and "friction-full."

A system that requires clinicians to manually compute a risk score is not sustainable. Models that automatically extract some predictors from the EHR but rely on the care team to enter others are probably doomed to failure. Instead, build the model based solely on factors that can be automatically extracted. Other important predictors that are not routinely recorded in the EHR can be added in a structured way and used prospectively. For example, an important AI tool may need patient data on BMI, exercise level, and smoking status and yet these are currently missing for most patients or are in an unusable text format. Restructure the intake form in the EHR to collect these variables and ensure more complete data on all patients. The key is engineering the environment for ease of use; for example, there are already a large number of online calculators, such as MDCalc (https://www.mdcalc.com/), which can be automated into the EHR or medical devices.

PRINCIPLE 45 • Form a small multidisciplinary collaborative <u>team</u> and meet regularly.

The ethical implementation of AI in health care requires that the workforce developing and implementing these tools be diverse. Team members may understand little about the work environments and pressures of the people from other fields and the metrics they use for measuring successful predictive models are often very different. Since team members need to be pulled from silos with different budgets and priorities, leaders need to ensure that these issues do not become obstacles.

So, the team must be <u>diverse</u> in multiple dimensions: race, gender, age, area of expertise, and profession and it needs a <u>Principal Investigator</u> who has protected time to devote to the project. Physician-scientists in a research fellowship are often ideal for this. If this person can be the dedicated implementation person, that is also helpful. If not, another member of the team must have sufficient protected time and motivation to fill the dedicated implementation role.

The team should ideally include experts from the clinical domain, biostatistics, machine learning, implementation/workflow science, senior mentors, stakeholders that will be affected from inside and outside the organization, and an ethicist. The biostatisticians are needed for the model development, evaluation, and the pragmatic study design and analysis. An experienced informatician is needed who has skill in exporting data and building models into the EHR—ideally, a dedicated person funded to work on your project who exports the correct data in the correct format for a statistical software package. Assembling this team is often a rate-limiting step, so it is important to get started early.

The team must have an experienced <u>project manager</u> who can identify project milestones and constraints. This person must be at a high level so that they have the ear of leaders. The ideal project manager has AI/statistical skills, can perform regulatory work (such as the Institutional Review Board applications and ClinicalTrials.gov documentation [https://clinicaltrials.gov/]), and can delegate work to others. The main goal of the project manager is to keep the project from floundering and make sure the right team members are meeting deadlines. The project manager must have enough experience and maturity to avoid making the project management a project in itself and must manage the full life cycle of the AI project.

It is just as important to keep the wrong people off the team. Avoid perfectionists, theoretical scientists, and those who are unpleasant to work with. Keep disruptive troublemakers off the team, which include those with a can't-do attitude and those who oppose change in general, or randomization and AI in particular. Develop a mechanism of removing people from the team who slow progress or annoy others. Leaders must be brave and address the problematic people who are obstacles to progress.

Each person on the team needs to bring their A-game and show that they have performed the work that they agreed to at the last meeting. If they do not, the other members can "encourage" forward progress. Teams that are successful find the right balance of collegiality and shared responsibility. Finally, the team needs senior, experienced mentors, who have a long-track record of success with similar projects.

A direct communication line to leaders who are responsive in the organization is needed. Leaders must ensure that the key stakeholders are supported and protected from encountering obstructionists who block forward progress.

The key is to build trusted relationships and find great partners to work with. Success requires that each team member learns from the others. This requires being empathic and patient enough to learn one another's terminology. It also requires curiosity and humbleness. The team must work together in a mutually beneficial relationship to align their goals.

PRINCIPLE 46 • Synergistic AI tools provide <u>clear explanations</u>. Algorithmic explicability is key to acceptance.

The AI user interface must make it clear "This patient is high risk because of A, B, and C." Minimize unnecessary black boxes (Figure 4.3). "Explainability," the ability to understand how an AI algorithm arrives at conclusions or predictions, is essential for AI success. Models should be transparent and allow users to see what factors create the probability (Figure 4.4). Black box models can be used—but are more challenging.

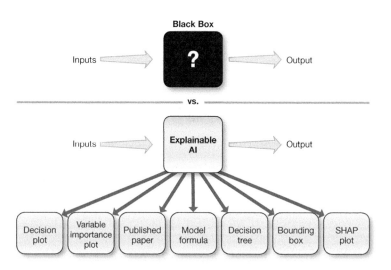

FIGURE 4.3. Model transparency vs black box models. A black box model is one that makes it difficult to impossible to understand how the inputs are converted to an output. Currently there are a large number of techniques for helping to explain these models.

VTE Risk Percentage (%)	Medication Group 1	Medication Group 2	DVT Indicator	Surgical Procedure Indicator	Cancer Indicator	Infectious Disease Indicator	Cardiology Indicator	Blood Gas Indicator	Central Line Indicator	Age (years)	MCHC	RDW CV Indicator	Lactate Indicator
77.0	X		X	X		X	X	X	X	6	X	X	X
66.5	X			X	X	X	X	X	X	19	X	X	X
34.5				X		X	X	X	X	2	X	X	X
29.8	X					X	X	X	X	19	X	X	X
27.7				X		X	X	X	X	1	X	X	X
28.9				X		X	X	X	X	1			
26.2				X		X	X	X	X	1	X	X	
27.9		X		X		X	X	X	X	6	X	X	X
25.9				X		X	X	X	X	1	X	X	X
27.4				X		X	X	X		1	X	X	X
25.3	X			X		X	X	X	X	1	X	X	X
26.3				X		X	X	X	X	1	X	X	
23.8				X		X	X	X	X	1	X	X	X
24.4	X			X				X	X	16	X	X	X
23.1		X		X			X	X	X	1	X	X	X
21.1				X		X	X	X	X	17	X	X	X

FIGURE 4.4. Example of a model providing real-time risk stratification. In this report, the probability of venous thromboembolism is displayed for all patients in the hospital. The model is explainable as the factors that drive the model are shown in the report. This report only shows the high-risk patients in the intervention half; the control group is not shown. This is a hypothetical version of a real report to protect patient confidentiality.

A *black box* refers to an AI tool or predictive model that offers little information regarding its logic operations and the critical elements that make it work. You can see the inputs and the output, but not the internal workings of the algorithm. In health care, black boxes require extra implementation effort. Numerous techniques are available to make this transparent, but clinicians are more likely to accept a model that is not a black box.

Clinical decision support in medicine should strive for transparency; however, some deep learning models, especially for high-dimensional data such as imaging, will be too complex to easily show what drives them. In this case, clinical care teams need to see evidence and validity to trust the model; they do not need to necessarily understand the black box. We trust Tylenol and anesthesia, even though we do not completely understand how they work. For example, in mammogram imaging analysis, the probability of breast cancer needs to be displayed but also the specific area of the mammogram that increased that probability needs to be identified (see Chapter 17). Once clinicians see demonstrations of the tools ability to predict against standard care, they will be more comfortable with the added information they provide to their own expertise.

To make a black box model more transparent, first ask "Who needs to know what?" A physician may not need to understand all of the weights for each node in neural network, but they may need to know the important drivers. Others may need to know information about the external validity or the statistical metrics. Others need a bounding box, which is simply a box or colored heatmap superimposed over an image to show the part of the image that is driving the prediction of cancer, for example. Sharing the right data with the right people makes the model less opaque which will improve its trustworthiness.

> *"The whole point of science is to open up black boxes, understand their insides, and build better boxes for the purposes of mankind."*
> —**BRAD EFRON**[16]

ℹ️ FOR MORE INFORMATION

Punish The Machine!: The Promise of Artificial Intelligence in Health Care. Uli Chettipally.[17]
Thinking, Fast and Slow, Deep Learning, and AI. Daniel Kahneman. Lex Fridman Podcast #65.[18]

CHAPTER SUMMARY

Successful clinician-computer partnerships require thoughtful implementation work and rigorous science to demonstrate the need for AI. Sustained acceptance requires that the interface is frictionless and adds value for both clinicians and patients but keeps the physician in the driver's seat. Health care leaders need to form and support multidisciplinary teams and function as catalysts to move projects along in the fragmented health care system. Statistical measures of performance are insufficient by themselves. The model metrics are proxies for what we really care about—improved patient health.

REFERENCES

1. Kumar A, Aikens RC, Hom J, et al. OrderRex clinical user testing: a randomized trial of recommender system decision support on simulated cases. *J Am Med Inf Assoc.* 2020;27(12):1850-1859.
2. Zhou Q, Chen ZH, Cao YH, Peng S. Clinical impact and quality of randomized controlled trials involving interventions evaluating artificial intelligence prediction tools: a systematic review. *NPJ Digit Med.* 2021;4(1):154.
3. Cabitza F, Rasoini R, Gensini GF. Unintended consequences of machine learning in medicine. *JAMA.* 2017;318(6):517-518.
4. Lyell D, Magrabi F, Raban MZ, et al. Automation bias in electronic prescribing. *BMC Med Inf Decis Making.* 2017;17(1):28.
5. Verghese A, Shah NH, Harrington RA. What this computer needs is a physician: humanism and artificial intelligence. *JAMA.* 2018;319(1):19-20.
6. Kahneman D. *Thinking, Fast and Slow.* Farrar, Straus and Giroux; 2011.
7. Chen JH, Asch SM. Machine learning and prediction in medicine—beyond the peak of inflated expectations. *N Engl J Med.* 2017;376(26):2507-2509.
8. Yiadom MYAB, Domenico HJ, Byrne DW, et al. Impact of a follow-up telephone call program on 30-day readmissions (FUTR-30): a pragmatic randomized controlled real-world effectiveness trial. *Med Care.* 2020;58(9):785-792.
9. Noto MJ, Domenico HJ, Byrne DW, et al. Chlorhexidine bathing and health care–associated infections: a randomized clinical trial. *JAMA.* 2015;313(4):369-378.
10. Hinton G. *Creative Destruction Lab. Machine Learning and the Market for Intelligence.* 2016; https://www.youtube.com/watch?v=2HMPRXstSvQ.
11. Susskind R, Susskind D. *The Future of the Professions: How Technology Will Transform the Work of Human Experts.* Oxford University Press; 2022.
12. Vasilevskis EE, Ouslander JG, Mixon AS, et al. Potentially avoidable readmissions of patients discharged to post-acute care: perspectives of hospital and skilled nursing facility staff. *J Am Geriatr Soc.* 2017;65(2):269-276.

13. Kripalani S, Roumie CL, Dalal AK, et al. Effect of a pharmacist intervention on clinically important medication errors after hospital discharge: a randomized trial. *Ann Intern Med*. 2012;157(1):1-10.

14. Bloom SL, Stollings JL, Kirkpatrick O, et al. Randomized clinical trial of an ICU recovery pilot program for survivors of critical illness. *Crit Care Med*. 2019;47(10):1337-1345.

15. Begoli E, Bhattacharya T, Kusnezov D. The need for uncertainty quantification in machine-assisted medical decision making. *Nat Mach Intell*. 2019;1:20-23.

16. Efron B. Comment on statistical modeling: the two cultures. *Stat Sci*. 2001; 16(3):218-219.

17. Chettipally UK. *Punish the Machine!: The Promise of Artificial Intelligence in Health Care*. Advantage Media Group; 2019.

18. Lex Fridman Podcast #65. *Daniel Kahneman: Thinking, Fast and Slow*. Deep Learning, and AI; 2020. https://www.youtube.com/watch?v=UwwBG-MbniY.

CHAPTER 5

Fairness—
Addressing the Ethical, Regulatory, and Privacy Issues

Many complex ethical issues surround the use of Artificial Intelligence (AI) in our society. In medicine, when AI models are improperly created, implemented, or evaluated, they are capable of leading to false conclusions, flawed clinical decision support, and can perpetuate inequities. This is a large and active area of research and numerous scholarly articles and links are listed below for further reading. The bottom line is that the key to progress in this area is using rigorous science to be evidence based so that AI tools improve health outcomes for all.

PRINCIPLE 47 • Don't break into jail. Be intentional about evaluating algorithms for bias, inequity, and potential harm.

Start with the assumption that the data, algorithms, and implementations of AI are problematic. Assume that the impact of AI will be unfair and that privacy problems will arise. Then collaborate with experts to use science and statistical analyses to discover ways to understand the biases and minimize inequity. Devote time and funding to ensuring that your AI tool not only addresses the minimum standard of fairness but breaks new ground in the science of AI fairness.

> *"One of the great things about AI is we should be able to use it both to identify disparities in healthcare and also to raise the standards of care for everybody."*
>
> —RUSS ALTMAN, STANFORD PROFESSOR OF BIOENGINEERING.

Bias can be introduced accidently through faulty models or by unknowingly implementing systems which systematically discriminate. So, time and resources must be set aside to discuss the assumptions of the AI model and develop appropriate solutions to potential problems.

There are many forms of bias that can lead to misunderstandings in these discussions. In science and statistics, the technical definition of bias is a systematic error in the data collected (statistic) compared with the truth (parameter). For example, self-reported age differs from the true computed age (today's date—date of birth) and it differs in a systematic way—an underestimate down to the whole number (always younger). This differs from random errors that could be underestimates or overestimates (younger or older). But complex racial and gender biases can be introduced and pose the most cause for concern. For example, suppose that an AI model provided bankers with advice on approving bank loans to customers. Let's assume that the AI algorithm included race as a predictor and did not clearly state how it performed calculations. As result of its use, the bank might be less likely to provide loans to applicants of a particular racial group—even if all other factors were the same. Unfair models like this implement predictors that systematically introduce bias, discriminate, and exclude. The recognition and replacement of unethical elements with appropriate predictors can improve AI tools. For example, race can be replaced with predictors that are a measure of the customer's loan repayment history. Care must be taken to not replace race with another proxy variable that is highly correlated with race, such as zip code. Care should be taken to avoid indirectly amplifying and perpetuating biases and errors in the data. For example, including health literacy in a model could introduce a bias that prevents patients with low literacy from receiving appropriate prevention measures. When AI tools are not carefully designed and evaluated, they can use and propagate bias. Yet, advancements have been made in recent years in the science of AI fairness that have shown that AI tools can be fairer and less biased than humans.

In another cautionary example, a paper published in *Science* showed that an AI tool designed to focus medical interventions on the sickest patients instead targeting resources on healthier White patients.[1] Scientific and statistical expertise is needed to assess for bias in the model, overall, and in various groups. The most important evaluation, however, is to test the impact of implementing a model, overall, and on vulnerable populations (Table 5.1).

The evaluations of bias must answer these questions:

What is the source of truth?
How was the original data set collected?
How is the data currently being collected?
Is the algorithm making assumptions?
Would implementation of the algorithm adversely impact a protected class or subgroup?
What evidence supports the conclusion that the AI system is fair?

TABLE 5.1	**Legally Recognized "Protected Classes" or "Sensitive Attributes" Based on U.S. Laws or Regulations[2]**

Race/ethnicity
Sex (including gender, sexual orientation, and gender identity).
Age
Physical or mental disability
Religion
National origin or ancestry
Citizenship
Pregnancy
Familial status
Veteran status

PRINCIPLE 48 • **The evaluation of AI fairness and equity must be ongoing during the entire project and is a process that is best managed with continuous quality improvement (CQI).**

Since AI fairness and equity issues are not an easy one-time fix, a CQI project provides the right framework.[3,4] The ethics of AI involves more than race and ethnicity. Ideally, each of the categories in Table 5.1 must be addressed. Also, strive to assess for fairness and equity by insurance type, income level, education level, etc. Therefore, these variables must be in your data dictionary, recorded and exported in your data set. The analyses can all be accomplished with sensitivity analysis that you put in the appendix of your paper. Willingness to adapt algorithms to improve fairness is essential. Although it is not feasible to address all these issues in any one project, this can be viewed as a long-term goal, which is why the CQI approach is ideal.[5]

PRINCIPLE 49 • **Avoid "colorblindness"—removal of race as a predictor is not a solution.[6]**

Be mindful of how the AI tool obtains, records, groups, and uses all variables that could be associated with protected and sensitive attributes. As we have seen, inappropriately including race in the model as a predictor could perpetuate unfair treatment or lack of treatment for communities of patients who have been systematically excluded and underserved.[7] Thoughtfully created predictive models can ensure that all patients who need a preventive intervention receive it—regardless of race. Again, in building AI tools, seek the advice of specialists to assess if there are biases that currently exist and then work with them to minimize carrying them forward.

> *"Rarely do we find men who are willing to engage in hard, solid thinking. There is an almost universal quest for easy answers and half-baked solutions. Nothing pains some people more than having to think."*
>
> —Rev. Dr. Martin Luther King, Jr
> (Strength to Love, 1963).

Models should be trained on a diverse population. Publication of predictive models should include a detailed Table 5.1 showing the diversity of the population and sensitivity analysis to assess how well the model performs overall and in diverse groups. Sensitivity analyses simply mean that the results are evaluated and displayed for subgroups. This *post hoc* analysis provides information about the robustness of the results and conclusions. The randomized controlled trial (RCT) should monitor how the model impacted outcomes in various groups. These issues must be studied, and the results transparently reported in papers. Of course, this requires having a sample that is large and diverse enough to provide meaningful conclusions from these subgroups. Not recording race and excluding race in all models is ignoring the problem, not solving it. This can be a challenge in some countries, such as Canada and France that do not routinely collect race in their electronic health record—or perhaps this is the better approach.

Our group created a predictive model of children with COVID-19 to estimate probability of requiring hospitalization.[8] Black and Hispanic/Latinx children with COVID-19 were more likely to require hospitalization. Leaving this factor out of the model could have resulted in Black and Hispanic children not being properly identified as high risk. In our paper, we provided two models: one with race and ethnicity and one without, allowing the user to decide which is appropriate in their situation. In many situations, if one can obtain a more comprehensive set of predictors directly related to the outcome, race may not be a significant predictor.

PRINCIPLE 50 • Involve stakeholders, including ethicists, data activists, patients and the public in the planning, execution, and reporting of the AI project.

Fairness and equity in AI are critical issues—not afterthoughts. The AI team must accept expert guidance from the communities that the system will affect and invests time and resources to do this appropriately; AI can, and will, be used in ways that are ethical and fair using deidentified data that are protecting personal information. Design the study and the analysis with a primary goal of minimizing inequity in "protected subgroups" (Table 5.1). Not recording (or exporting data on) these variables and "forbidding" these variables as predictors and features in AI algorithms are not effective approaches. The solution is to ensure that measures of health are improved even as methods are automated at scale—overall, and in these protected groups.

Therefore, it is wise to include a community advisory board, an ethicist, patients, and others potentially impacted downstream on the team and data and safety monitoring committees. Consider using one of the three specific aims in a National Institutes of Health grant for the study of these issues. A bioethicist can be partially funded for this work to address the topics in Table 5.2 with more nuanced solutions.

TABLE 5.2	The Elements of Fair and Responsible AI

1. Ethical purpose—How will it benefit patients and society?
2. Accountability—Who is responsible for the way it works?
3. Transparency—How was the model developed and how will it be implemented?
4. Explainability—How does the algorithm work to convert inputs to outputs?
5. Fairness and nondiscrimination—Is the model helping all groups?
6. Safety and reliability—Is the model harmless and stable?
7. Open and fair competition—Has the model been compared to alternative approaches?
8. Privacy—How has the confidential patient data been protected?
9. Robustness—Is the model empirically sound in different locations and across time?
10. Beneficence—Is the model benefiting patients?
11. Nonmaleficence—Has there been research to assess harm to or neglect of patients?
12. Autonomy—Have patients been informed about decisions affecting their medical care?
13. Justice—Is there a fair and equitable distribution of burden and resources?

PRINCIPLE 51 • Develop internal and external communications to address concerns that patients have about AI and measure progress over time.

Many patients are concerned that AI will replace their doctor (Table 5.3). The message should be "We are listening to your concerns about the use of AI and have solutions." Many doctors, especially radiologists and dermatologist, are concerned that AI will replace them. Projects need to show how AI can help by augmenting prediction and providing clinical decision support but not substitution. The exception to this could occur in countries with a shortage of medical specialists, but even in these countries the AI is not replacing a specialist, it is providing specialist-level expertise to primary care physicians and other providers who otherwise lack this expertise.

Do not dismiss these concerns. The involvement of key stakeholders in the planning, development, and execution of AI tools is vital to fairness. Patients will be concerned that AI is targeting them or tracking them. Communicate how the model is specifically designed to include variables believed to contribute to better health for all patients. Through clear documentation and a communication plan, resistance will be lowered, and you will empower patients with knowledge from the AI tool. Patients want to know and be involved in their own care. Let the patients and clinicians know that a model is being used in their care.

TABLE 5.3	Concerns From the Public About Using AI in Medicine

"I don't want to have the computer making decisions instead of my doctor."
"My privacy may not be protected."
"The AI technology is not mature enough for medical applications."
"I don't trust the AI companies."
"What about my choice as a patient?"
"Will the model target or track me?"
"Will this increase my health care costs?"
"The data are probably biased."
"Will my data be shared without my knowledge?"
"This could widen the digital divide."
"AI could exacerbate existing racial disparities."

PRINCIPLE 52• Be transparent and document steps taken to improve AI fairness.

Not only does the AI tool need to improve outcomes in patients (overall and in these protected classes), but the algorithm must also be transparent and flexible—especially in a real-world health care setting. The ideal way to be transparent is to form a plan to disseminate the information to the public and publish papers in high-profile medical journals with a detailed appendix. Dissemination to the patients and public is accomplished in print, digitally, and in video and new research is now showing which methods work best for different situations.[9]

Variables, such as sex and gender, must be thoughtfully recorded and considered as predictors. Automatically omitting sex and gender from AI tools is not the solution.

Men and women suffering from a heart attack report different symptoms in an emergency department. Ignoring gender in an AI tool to compute probability of a heart attack would be foolish. AI should be optimized to use variables that are significant for all people. This needs to be part of the evaluation. Are there unintended consequences of including gender identity in a model? Do all subgroups show improvement? Are there subgroups that are harmed by this? Is there an age-gender interactions that could be used as a predictor to improve the outcome for all groups?

How will you document that you have addressed these ethical issues? In the appendix of your paper, report model performance metrics, such as the receiver-operating-characteristic and calibration curves for these subgroups, and then include a forest plot showing the impact of the model for these subgroups. See Chapter 3 for more detail.

PRINCIPLE 53• Learn how to rigorously assess a model for bias. (Table 5.4)

TABLE 5.4	How to Assess a Model for Bias

Assess the area under the receiver-operating-characteristic curve for each protected class or subgroup, plot the receiver-operating-characteristic and calibration curves.

Create a model for each protected class or subgroup and compare results.

(continued)

TABLE 5.4 *Continued*

Assess the association between protected class and the predictors in the model.

Create a model to predict a protected class from the predictors and the end point in the model.

Create a spline graph of the given prevention treatment on y vs probability of the outcomes on x, with lines for protected classes.

Create a spline graph of the outcome on y vs probability of the outcomes on x, with lines for protected classes.

Create a forest plot of the impact of the model on the protected classes.

Perform uncertainty quantification for subgroups and protected classes. Are there groups for which the 95% confidence interval is just too wide?

Create a classification and regression tree overall and for various protected classes to understand the model performance.

Use explainable AI techniques to help solve bias issues.

Finally, document and share with others your work in this area. Include a section in your paper or appendix showing your analysis of this work to minimize inequities in protected classes.

PRINCIPLE 54• Challenge the model.

Researchers can purposely create a biased model and using simulation analyses learn how to recognize and debias a real model.

Experiment by taking a real data set and introducing artificial biases (none, small, medium, strong). Test how it would change the model and outcome. Ask: how could we detect bias with real data? Ask: are there any interactions of subgroups on outcome?

Conduct research to understand potential biases. For example, create one model for Group A and one for Group B and compare them. What would be the implications of implementing these models? Assess what would happen if the implementation of the models were switched for these groups.

Analyze the data set to see if any racial group was underdiagnosed or treated in a biased way. Assess for interactions between race and the predictors and race and the outcome. More research is needed to understand and improve fairness and equity with simulation studies. For example, the data can be manipulated to show that wealthy insured patients are coded to receive the best treatment options resulting in the best outcomes, while poor uninsured patients are coded to receive only the basic treatment options resulting in poor outcomes. How would you detect that with a real data set?

Include a social determinant of health in the model as a predictor. Does it perpetuate bias? What are the understood socio-economic factors that indirectly capture, imply, or perpetuate the bias? Test these variables to understand their impact. All of these potential forms of bias need to be compared in the pragmatic RCT, to the parallel control group.

PRINCIPLE 55 • Use <u>federated learning</u> and other modern techniques for external validation.

> *"A promising method for permitting data use involves "behind the glass" access for outside parties so that data don't leave the institution."*

—Kenneth Mandl, and Eric Perakslis.[10]

Health data privacy issues are important and need to be addressed in a fair and balanced way.[10] Federated learning (or collaborative learning) is a collaborative AI technique used to create and validate models by storing the data on multiple servers with the local samples, without exchanging the data between groups or combining the data sets on one computer. For example, three hospitals could store their own data on their computer systems and provide the AI creator remote access to fit a model remotely without transferring the data out of that hospital's computer system. This approach can solve an important problem—many AI models need larger and more diverse data sets, but the organizations that own the data sets are reluctant or unable to exchange confidential patient data. The patient data never leave the home institution, only the model characteristics are shared. Successfully implementing this approach will require more funding and research but it has great potential.[11]

For external validation of models, there are concerns about institutions sharing patient data sets. If using a federated learning approach, the model formula, with the coefficients/parameters, can be shared. This enables others to assess the external validity of a model without sharing any data. In fact, this information should be included in the appendix of most papers about AI and predictive models.

Another method of collaborating without transferring confidential data is to have collaborators fund part of your biostatistician's effort for analysis. This way the data remain at the home institution, but collaborators can have analyses performed, test various models, and coauthor papers efficiently. Sometimes people do not need to share data—they need to share knowledge about the model.

PRINCIPLE 56 • **In many cases, it is <u>unethical to NOT randomize</u> and NOT learn which approach provides the best overall health results.**

Attempting to stop AI projects until there are no biases in the data is unrealistic. Yet, there is a possibility that AI tools could worsen outcomes for patients or for subgroups if scientific rigor is not used in AI evaluations. Here randomization can be justified from a safety perspective. As discussed in Chapter 3, one strategy is to phase AI tools in slowly and assess if there is more benefit than harm through RCT design. Rigorous science will enable us to adopt AI in health care at the optimal pace—not too fast and not too slow.

Do not overpromise the benefits of AI in medicine. False claims can be a deceptive act or practice that has legal ramifications.

AI has amazing potential in medicine, but some of the declarations of victory have been premature. AI entrepreneurs and enthusiasts are optimistic but claims that exaggerate the capability of AI risk falling into the category of "deceptive practices" by the U.S. Federal Trade Commission (FTC). Racially biased algorithms can now also fall in this category. "The FTC Act prohibits unfair or deceptive practices. That would include the sale or use of, eg, racially biased algorithms."[12]

ℹ️ FOR MORE INFORMATION

Algorithmovigilance—Advancing Methods to Analyze and Monitor Artificial Intelligence–Driven Health Care for Effectiveness and Equity. Peter Embi.[6]
AI at Historically Black Colleges and Universities.[13]
AI and analytics from an HBCU perspective.[14]
The Ethical Algorithm. Kearns and Roth.[15]
Group fairness and individual fairness. Mikhail Yurochkin.[16]
Invisible Women: Data Bias in a World Designed for Men. Caroline Criado Perez.[17]
The Pursuit of Wow! Tom Peters.[3]
The Man Who Discovered Quality. Andrea Gabor.[4]
MIT OpenCourseWare. Machine Learning for Healthcare. Regulation of Machine Learning/Artificial Intelligence in the US. Andy Coravos, Mark Shervey.[18]
MIT OpenCourseWare. Machine Learning for Healthcare. Fairness. Peter Szolovits.[19]
Introduction to Deep Learning. Lecture 8. AI Bias and Fairness. Ava Soleimany.[20]

CHAPTER SUMMARY

We are all responsible for minimizing inequities related to AI in medicine and therefore we must search out potential causes of bias and address them. The patients and clinicians affected need to be included in the design and implementation of the tools. Bioethicists are needed on the AI team.

The goals of responsible implementation of AI in medicine are to (1) improve health overall, (2) improve health in protected classes, and (3) to minimize inequality in outcomes. Prospective RCTs provide the facts about health impact and are therefore the best approach to accomplish these goals.

Excluding variables of protected classes from data collection, models, and sensitivity analysis can be counterproductive. Responsible AI requires that clinical experts lead, remain in the decision loop, review the AI results, and combine this with other information to make a fair and balanced decision. The onus of informing the patients and those involved in their care is on the AI team and administration. Trust and adoption of AI requires dissemination of information about tool design, implementation, and findings. If we do this wrong, AI will amplify biases in society. If we do this right, AI will reduce biases.

REFERENCES

1. Obermeyer Z, Powers B, Vogeli C, Mullainathan S. Dissecting racial bias in an algorithm used to manage the health of populations. *Science*. 2019;366(6464):447-453.
2. Barocas S, Hardt M. Fairness in machine learning. NIPS 2017 Tutorial—Part I. https://fairmlbook.org/tutorial1.html.
3. Peters T. *The Pursuit of Wow! Every Person's Guide to Topsy-Turvy Times*. Vintage; 1994.
4. Gabor A. *The Man Who Discovered Quality: How W. Edwards Deming Brought the Quality Revolution to America*. Penguin Books; 1992.
5. Smith M, Sattler A, Hong G, Lin S. From code to bedside: implementing artificial intelligence using quality improvement methods. *J Gen Intern Med*. 2021;36(4):1061-1066.
6. Embi PJ. Algorithmovigilance-advancing methods to analyze and monitor artificial intelligence-driven health care for effectiveness and equity. *JAMA Netw Open*. 2021;4(4):e214622.
7. Vyas DA, Eisenstein LG, Jones DS. Hidden in plain sight—reconsidering the use of race correction in clinical algorithms. *N Engl J Med*. 2020;383(9):874-882.

8. Howard LM, Garguilo K, Gillon J, et al. The first 1000 symptomatic pediatric SARS-CoV-2 infections in an integrated health care system: a prospective cohort study. *BMC Pediatr.* 2021;21(1):403.

9. Cook S, Mayers S, Goggins K, et al. Assessing research participant preferences for receiving study results. *J Clin Transl Sci.* 2019;4(3):243-249.

10. Mandl KD, Perakslis ED. HIPAA and the leak of "deidentified" EHR data. *N Engl J Med.* 2021;384(23):2171-2173.

11. Rieke N, Hancox J, Li W, et al. The future of digital health with federated learning. *NPJ Digit Med.* 2020;3:119.

12. Jillson E. *Aiming for Truth, Fairness, and Equity in Your Company's Use of AI.* 2021. https://www.ftc.gov/business-guidance/blog/2021/04/aiming-truth-fairness-equity-your-companys-use-ai

13. AI at historically black colleges and universities. https://charlescearl.github.io/ai-hbcu/

14. AI and analytics from an HBCU perspective. https://www2.deloitte.com/us/en/pages/technology/articles/ai-and-analytics-from-an-hbcu-perspective.html

15. Kearns M, Roth A. *The Ethical Algorithm—The Science of Socially Aware Algorithm Design.* Oxford University Press; 2019.

16. Yurochkin M, Bower A, Sun Y. *International Conference on Learning Representations;* 2020. *Training individually fair ML models with sensitive subspace robustness.* https://arxiv.org/abs/1907.00020

17. Perez C. *Invisible Women: Data Bias in a World Designed for Men.* Harry N. Abrams; 2021.

18. Coravos A, Shervey M. MIT OpenCourseWare. Regulation of machine learning/artificial intelligence in the US. https://www.youtube.com/watch?v=k95abdkdCPk

19. Szolovits P. MIT OpenCourseWare. Machine learning for healthcare. Fairness. https://www.youtube.com/watch?v=zYgkr0KfWM0

20. Soleimany A. Introduction to deep learning. Lecture 8. AI Bias and Fairness. https://www.youtube.com/watch?v=wmyVODy_WD8

The Mechanics

6

Modeling—
An Overview of
Predictive Modeling,
Neural Networks,
and Deep Learning

Although Artificial Intelligence (AI) can provide very accurate predictions in medicine, the predictions about AI in medicine have been wildly inaccurate. The progress of AI over time is illustrated in Figure 6.1. From its inception in 1956 until the middle of the 1990s, progress was stagnant.

"Deep learning is going to be able to do everything."
—**Geoffrey Hinton, (2020).**

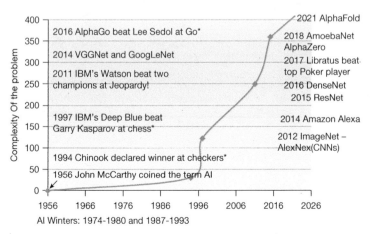

FIGURE 6.1. Progress of AI over time. The work in AI today is at a really profound level. A few milestones are plotted here with the Y-axis equal to the game-tree complexity (log base 10) for the milestones marked with an asterisk, while others are based on the year accomplished.

101

In the past 2 decades, we have seen explosive growth in the ability of AI to master more and more complex problems. Yet, for the most part, these advances have not made their way into health care. Table 6.1 illustrates some of the reasons why.

> *"We tend to overestimate the effect of a technology in the short run and underestimate the effect in the long run."*
>
> —Amara's law. (Roy Amara).

TABLE 6.1	Challenges of Implementing AI in Health Care
Traditional AI works in these settings	**AI struggles to work in health care**
Simple rules (chess)	Complex rules (human body)
Facts (Jeopardy!)	Debates (medical and scientific literature)
High signal:noise (Go)	Low signal:noise (PubMed, electronic health record)
Unbiased data (rules, facts, winners, and losers)	Biased data (publication bias, confounding by indication, and many other forms of bias)
Stakes are low (games)	Stakes are high (lives depend on the answer)
Easy to implement (a competition)	Complex to implement (a randomized controlled trial in a hospital)

PRINCIPLE 57 • **Prioritize AI Projects by Likelihood of Success.**

TABLE 6.2	Questions to Assess the Likelihood of an AI Pragmatic Trial's Success

1. Can the primary end point (an important patient outcome) be ascertained in routine care?
2. If implemented as planned, will this AI project improve an important patient outcome?
3. Will it help accomplish an organizational goal?
4. If the outcome is predicted, is there agreement to make prevention or treatment actionable?
   a. Is there support for implementation from the hospital operations groups?
   b. Does the project have a leader and team that will make it likely to be successful?
5. Is it technically feasible to predict the outcome with AI?
6. Is there wide variability in the results that clinicians provide currently?
7. Are the sample size and event rate large enough to detect a statistically significant improvement?
8. Do we have the funding to pay for this?
9. If successful, is it likely to lower cost or result in a fundable grant?

PRINCIPLE 58 • **Create an AI Playbook for Each Project.**

In football, the coach develops a strategy of plays or tactics to win the game. Create a strategic plan like this for the success of your model from start to finish (Tables 6.2 and 6.3).

PRINCIPLE 59 • **Create a data dictionary to define a data set with a comprehensive list of potential predictors from a wide range of domains and then let the data teach you which are the most important.**

A data dictionary is a document, often a spreadsheet, that specifies a collection of variables from a database, such as the electronic health record (EHR). AI researchers will create a data dictionary of the potential predictors and outcomes that they are interested in exporting for a model (Table 6.4). The purpose is to create a single source of truth that can be replicated. The dictionary not only

TABLE 6.3	Playbook for Creating and Testing an AI Tool

1. Choose a feasible study based on the questions in Table 6.2.
2. Identify a finite problem to solve—not the cure for cancer.
3. Find a clinical leader who has the expertise and free time to make the project a success. For example, a research fellow with a good mentor.
4. Form a team based on the recommendations in this book.
5. Create a data dictionary of the variables to export. Include variables that are clinically important and those that have been used in previous scoring systems and models (Table 6.4).
6. Assess if the model is biased or unfair. Test and modify.
7. Institutional Review Board approval to export a data set.
8. Export a comprehensive data set in a clean flat file that can be analyzed. Obtain a data set of the outcome and as many potential predictors as possible.
9. Perform data cleaning and management. Debug your data before you debug your model.
10. Divide your data so that you can perform an external temporal validation, for example, into the early 80% (data set A) and the later 20% (data set B).
11. Study the TRIPOD guidelines and create a plan to follow them.
12. Create a flowchart for how you will create your model. This will be in the appendix of your paper.
13. Test the predictors in data set A against the outcome in a uni-variate fashion.
14. Build a model according to your prespecified plan.
15. Perform an external temporal validation in data set B. Publish a paper about the model.
16. Code the model into the electronic health record.
17. Write a protocol for the pragmatic randomized controlled trial and include an adaptive platform aspect.
18. Obtain Institutional Review Board approval with waiver of consent to randomize patients to usual care vs usual care + the model.
19. Register it with https://clinicaltrials.gov/
20. Run it silently in the background
21. Get leadership and front-line support for the effector arm strategy of focusing prevention based on high risk in a random half.

TABLE 6.3	*Continued*

22. Create an alert and a system to triple check that prevention is performed on high risk.
23. Focus the prevention/intervention on the high-risk patients.
24. Assess safety and efficacy with a data and safety monitoring board
25. Analyze the results. Test if the system improves health outcomes.
26. If yes, turn model on for all. If no, move to phase 2 of your adaptive platform trial.
27. Publish a paper describing the impact of the model in a high-profile journal to teach others.
28. Find collaborators to perform geographical validations.

TABLE 6.4	**Potential Predictor Variables for the Data Dictionary**

Commonly used predictors (Table 6.5) and predictors used in similar models

Published risk factors

Demographic data and variables needed for the paper's Table 1 (age, sex, etc)

Variables to assess bias, protected classes. (See Table 5.1)

Laboratory data (complete blood count, basic metabolic panel, arterial blood gases)

Factors that will be important for sensitivity analyses

Identifiers for longitudinal follow-up (first, middle, and last name, social security number, date of birth, gender, race, marital status, last known state of residence, state of birth, age at death, state of death, date or year of death, date of last contact, and father's surname)

Psychosocial variables

Variables that reviewers may ask about—potential confounders

Electronic health record (EHR) audit logs which measure users' interactions with the patients (orders, messages, flowsheets, chart review notes, and general documentation)

Epic user-EHR interaction categories

Historical ICD diagnosis codes, which can be mapped to phenome-wide association study codes (Phecodes).

Genetic data

includes the variable name, but also the variable label/description and a reproducible definition to extract the field from a database. The data dictionary also specifies the data type—integer, date, or string text. Many variables are repeated and therefore careful instructions about which variable to extract are important, for example, the first on admission, the highest, the lowest, or the last in a series.

To support the reproducibility at another institution, especially for the outcome variable, take care to ensure that the data dictionary provides enough detail. Many projects require merging data sets from different sources; the data dictionary should specify unique identifiers that can be used for merging. Blood tests that are performed in panels, such as the complete blood count, can be requested by the panel instead of individually. This requires little extra work and can be valuable in your model creation. A technique for improving models is to identify the top three strongest predictors and then work to export variables that capture more detail around those predictors. For example, if "smoker" was known to be a strong predictor, capture pack-years and other details to quantitate smoking. Finally, the team should have one master copy of the data dictionary in a shared folder or drive.

PRINCIPLE 60 • Choose model variables which have a known and valid source of truth. The variables should be structured, captured accurately across all patients, and be consistently recorded.

What do you do if a predictor is important but missing for many patients? For example, albumin is the second strongest predictor of pressure injuries (after the Braden Scale) but is missing for about 80% of patients in the hospital. After extensive statistical analysis of the various approaches, we found that using the median albumin value for those with a missing value works well and is feasible in a real-time predictive model. More complex methods of assessing the missing value, such as multiple imputation, give similar results but make it impossible to use in practice for real-time predictive models.

If a predictor has missing information, replacing the missing with the median value works well in most cases and is feasible. More complex approaches can make it impossible to implement and often do not add value.

One issue that arises in building predictive models from the EHR data is how to handle predictors that are not 100% perfect. The reality is that if the imperfect predictor improves your model, then it should be useful prospectively in a real-time model. The outcome variable, however, does require rigorous validation. This can be performed with a chart audit of a random sample. Reviewers will be very focused on your precise definition of the outcome variable and how reproducible it is.

Avoid building models using complete-case analyses. This method excludes all patients who are missing any of the predictors in the model. This can lead to very misleading conclusions and biased models. For example, if you create a predictive model that uses one of the variables from an arterial blood gas test and use complete-case analysis, your model will be based on the subset of the most critically ill patients in the hospital. In the appendix of your paper, you can provide more detail about how you handled missing data, for example, multiple imputation, sensitivity, and tipping point analysis.

Social determinants of health, and both literacy and numeracy, clearly impact health. They are often proposed as ways to improve predictive models in health care, but they can be problematic. First, these variables are not routinely captured and recorded in a structured routine method at most hospitals and therefore are not useful for tools that are designed to work at many institutions. Second, they rarely improve the performance of models once the variables in Table 6.5 are included. Third, their inclusion can cause ethical problems if they are indirectly correlated with subgroups and protected classes. For example, even if one leaves race out of a model but includes social determinants of health, the model can indirectly use race as a predictor, which may cause unintended ethical problems.

PRINCIPLE 61 • Keep an open mind about using a wide range of predictor variables.

Many of the previous failures in AI were related to researchers overemphasizing the importance of the "predictor" they were studying in isolation of all other predictors. Genetic researchers exaggerate the contribution of genetics. Biomarker researchers exaggerate the importance of their biomarkers. Success requires keeping an open mind about the relative importance of predictors and using the predictors that are the strongest and most feasible to use—even if they are not the most novel.

A good example of this is predicting type 2 diabetes. Although there are hundreds of papers on the association of genetics on the development of diabetes, body mass index (BMI) is a stronger predictor. BMI alone outperforms the genetic information combined in a genome-wide association study. Once the BMI is accounted for, the genetic information generally does not improve upon the prediction.[1] So, in building an AI tool for risk of diabetes, obviously BMI would be the better predictor because it is free and available for everyone simply by asking two questions: height and weight. Genetics alone is not the solution to personalized medicine AI tools. For many conditions, the proportion of outcome explained by genetics is small and sometimes exaggerated. The solution is to be objective and open-minded about the strength of predictors and includes a wide range of predictor variables.

TABLE 6.5	List of Commonly Used Predictors in Health Care Predictive Models for Consideration in the Data Dictionary (Sorted by Level of Importance)

Age
Body mass index
Sex/gender
Smoking status
Blood pressure
Exercise level
Red cell distribution width
Medications
Cholesterol
Diabetes
Blood urea nitrogen
Glucose
Albumin
Stress level
Chloride
Carbon dioxide
Platelet count
White blood cell count
Race/ethnicity
Job satisfaction
Hematocrit
Hemoglobin
Calcium
Happiness level
Cancer diagnosis

PRINCIPLE 62 • **Most predictive models are designed to identify which patients are at high risk, but the goal is not to change the predictors. AI tools that attempt to both identify the high-risk patient and determine the treatment plan often fail.**

The goal of the predictive model is to predict and provide accurate and precise granular risk stratification, not to solve the problem, not to recommend how to alter the predictors to change the patients risk level. Models should not be limited to predictors that are actionable. The purpose of the model is to identify the high-risk patients. The needed intervention for the patient at high risk is a different issue. Occasionally, one might choose to create a predictive model in which all of the predictors are actionable, but this is an unusual situation. More commonly a model is created that can identify the patients at high risk. For example, age and sex are in most risk stratification models, but the intention is never to modify these factors. The health care system's interventions to prevent the outcome are usually unrelated to the predictors.

PRINCIPLE 63 • When assessing potential variables for inclusion in a model be an objective scientist and apply modern statistical skills.

The rigid old-school approach of statistical predictive modeling is one in which medical domain experts define the predictors and the statistician does not deviate from those when creating a model. This outdated approach does not work for AI. While one begins by assessing the potential predictors that the experts agree are important, understand that their list may be incomplete and there may be false assumptions. For our work in predictive modeling of readmissions, the experts held that the following factors would predict 30-day hospital readmission: uninsured status, low literacy, certain psychosocial variables, and socioeconomic status factors. In that analysis, none of those factors were accurate predictors of the likelihood of readmission, while other predictors, such as the red cell distribution width (RDW), were and were not on anyone's radar. Surprisingly, RDW turned out to be important in many predictive models.[2,3]

PRINCIPLE 64 • One can build a predictive model based on factors known within the first 24 hours and update the probability each day.

For a predictive model to be useful in a hospital setting, the model must be able to form a prediction based on variables that are available on admission—or at least within the first 24 hours. Subsequently, this model needs to update each day to provide the latest probability. We found that it was useful to display both the admission probability and the current probability in the EHR allowing clinicians to see the changes. Our approach is to use the same model and update it with new data each day. Some have argued that it would be better to export a data set from days 2, 3, 4, etc, and create new models with new predictors and coefficients for each day. This is unnecessary and not feasible. This type of perfectionist thinking causes paralysis of projects.

As with the weather forecast, there is a "horizon effect" in modeling. In this effect, the model becomes more accurate as one gets closer to the event. While a patient is in the hospital, it can be helpful to have predictive models of what will happen after discharge, for example, a blood clot. As the length of stay becomes shorter, these models are becoming more and more important.

PRINCIPLE 65 • **Use the "Domenico Guidelines" to narrow your potential predictors to form a robust model. Use a modern and reproducible technique to select predictors for a model.**

To create a model in the most robust way that would satisfy reviewers at high-profile journals and meet the TRIPOD reporting standards, my colleague, Henry Domenico, a Lead Biostatistician at Vanderbilt University Medical Center, developed the guidelines in Table 6.6.

TABLE 6.6	The Domenico Guidelines—Basic Approach to Model Building and Validation

1. Carefully define the outcome, unit of analysis, how the model will be used, and when predictions need to be made available.
2. Conduct a literature review and consult with the domain experts. Develop a list of candidate predictors. Also identify variables that will be needed for Table 1 and subgroup analyses. Refine the candidate predictor list to those that meet criteria for how the model will be used. Discuss how race and ethnicity will be treated in the model. Remove variables that could have a reverse-causal relationship with the outcome.
3. Consider interactions and nonlinear effects. Specify these in a candidate variable list. Consider how discrete variables will be grouped. Avoid unnecessary dichotomization of continuous variables.
4. Consider how missing data will be handled both in model building and in practice.
5. Consider how validation will be performed. If enough events, set aside recent subset for temporal external validation. If not enough events, specify internal validation methods to be used (bootstrap, leave-one-out cross validation, etc).

TABLE 6.6	*Continued*

6. Using historical data, rate estimates, or observed data prior to model, determine or approximate the actual number of events that will be used for modeling.

7. Ensure that number of events is sufficient to support the model including full candidate list (events per degrees of freedom ≥20). If events/degrees of freedom are less than 20, refer to Van Smeden paper.[4] May need to remove potential variables from candidate list; remove nonlinearity, or remove interactions.

8. Fit a logistic regression model using all candidate predictors.

9. Test for multicollinearity using Variance Inflation Factors. Remove variables as needed. The model at this point is referred to as the "full model."

10. Remove variables, interaction terms, and nonlinear effect terms with a non-significant contribution to model using ANOVA chi-square criteria. Specify a priori variables that will remain in model regardless of the results from this step.

11. Refit model after nonsignificant factors are removed. The model at this step is referred to as the "reduced model."

12. Compare internal calibration metrics of full and reduced models:
    - Calibration curves
    - Area under the receiver-operating-characteristic curve, Brier score
    - Bootstrap calibration slope and intercept
    - Scatterplot of reduced vs full model predicted values

13. If no substantial reduction in predictive accuracy, designate reduced model as the primary model.

14. Test the primary model in validation dataset or using other validation technique.

15. Fit any alternative AI or ML models using the full pool of candidate predictors. Compare performance to the full and reduced logistic models in both model development and validation cohorts. Validation cohort performance is the most important factor to consider. Weigh any improvement in performance against added model complexity.

16. Test model performance within subgroups emphasizing populations at risk for unanticipated harm.

PRINCIPLE 66 • Learn the most popular analytic methods.

Many are surprised that the most popular AI technique among data scientists is logistic regression, followed by decision trees and gradient booting machines. The most commonly used inferential statistical techniques in modern medical research can be found in Table 16.1 in Publishing Your Medical Research and on slide 48 at SlideShare.[5]

Before implementing a complex model with many predictor variables/features, check that a simpler model would not work as well. Even if the complex model buys you a little bit extra in the area under the receiver-operating-characteristic curve (AUC), if it is not explainable and cannot be implemented in practice, it is not the better option.

Avoid circular logic errors caused by predictors that are based on reverse causation.

Complex models may initially appear to be superior to a simpler logistic regression model but when one "looks under the hood" it becomes clear that the model is not superior and at times fatally flawed. This can result from reverse causation, predictors that could not be used in practice, or other problems. Reverse causation means that an outcome variable is used as a predictor.

With traditional statistical model building, one needs subject matter expertise and biostatistical expertise to jointly think about the advantages and disadvantage of using various potential predictors. When was that variable recorded? What is the cause-effect relationship? Is it logical that this variable could predict this outcome? With machine learning (ML) some believe that neither is really needed because a large number of predictors/features can be used without a concern of overfitting. This automation can lead to using variables to predict the outcome which are nonsensical. For example, an ML model was designed to predict which hospital patients were most likely to die. The model was a black box, meaning it was difficult to understand what the predictors were. In fact, if the patient was visited by the chaplain, the model "predicted" the patient would die.[6,7]

Below are some examples of **accidently fitting confounders** rather than including variables that offer a true signal. This means that a predictive model is created that used "predictors" that are just another way of describing the outcome:

A ruler in a pathology image next to a skin lesion "predicts" cancer.
"Urgent" on X-ray "predicts" a hip fracture.
Patients with more potential predictors/features were more likely to develop
    depression.

A medication used to treat sepsis is used to "predict" sepsis.

A chest tube to treat a pneumothorax is used to "predict" it.

A red circle around a lung tumor on a chest X-ray is used to "predict" lung cancer.

Because ML neural networks are black boxes, "predictors" like those listed above—for example, a red circle—can become part of a model. These models have good statistical performance but obviously do not perform well in practice. Be very skeptical of a model that performs too well and review for reverse causation. Recognizing reverse causation is an important AI skill.

> *"Biology at its most fundamental level is an information processing system."*
>
> —Demis Hassabis, CEO of DeepMind.

PRINCIPLE 67 • Understand the differences between the learning categories of AI.

1. **Supervised Learning**—an approach to creating AI models in which the algorithm is attempting to use inputs to predict a labeled output category. For example, patients are categorized (labeled), as cancer or benign and then a model is created to predict cancer from demographic data, laboratory data, and an X-ray.

2. **Unsupervised Learning**—an approach to creating AI models in which the algorithm is attempting to cluster cases into meaningful groups. Patients are not categorized by humans and instead the model tries to define important subtypes or clusters. For example, a large data set of lupus patients might be used to understand important subtypes.

3. **Deep Reinforcement Learning** (RL)—an approach to creating AI models in which the algorithm is attempting to use feedback it receives from various attempts to become better and better at a game or another system. In this form of ML, an "agent" learns how to take "actions" to maximize a total "reward."[8] The algorithm will try something, and the system will reward or punish it. This process is repeated many times to develop actions that lead to the most rewards. This approach has been used to develop models for games, but this is now being used in medicine. One group recently used RL to study anticoagulant treatment recommendations for patients with atrial fibrillation and the impact on outcomes.[8]

PRINCIPLE 68 • Explore several different modeling techniques for their strengths and weaknesses. Then present the complete performance of each model for others to compare.

One of the problems holding AI back is that many AI researchers understand and prefer one approach, which they use for all problems. A more effective approach is to be agnostic and open-minded about the various tools. An important point here is to compare not only the AUC but also the calibration and other metrics for both the training and validation data sets. Some methods appear to be an improvement in the AUC but then the calibration graphs show real problems in the performance.

For example, you might compare the following approaches. Show the pros and cons of each to the reviewers and readers and explain why you settled on one technique for your application.

1. Logistic regression
2. Random forest
3. Deep learning
4. XGBoost

The major categories of AI can be grouped as follows:

Statistical models/regression

Logistic Regression—this is one of the most popular and powerful methods of creating predictive models for binary end points. The advantages of logistic regression are that it provides robust models that are easy to understand and implement into the EHR. Logistic models do not require massive data sets to build and can be built with 15 events (outcomes) per variable. The disadvantage is that logistic regression it is not suitable for high-dimensional data such as medical images, speech, or electrocardiograms.

Once we have a logistic regression model, we take the weights (betas) and convert them into an equation that provides a probability. We will start with the simplest model with one predictor. Let's take a simple example: preventing pressure injuries (ulcers, bedsores) in hospitalized patients. Suppose that we wanted to create a predictive model of pressure injury from the Braden Scale. The formula would look like this: $Z = $ intercept $+$ beta1 x Braden_Scale. Probability of a pressure injury $= 1/(1 + e^{-Z})$ where $e = 2.718$. The more complete model looks like this: $Z = $ intercept $+$ beta1 $\times$ Braden_Scale $+$ beta2 $\times$ albumin, etc.

Machine learning

Neural networks are a form of AI that takes inputs, weights them, passes them on to the next layer, and then outputs a prediction of the answer. The approach is based on a simplified version of how the human brain functions (Figure 6.2).

Chapter 19 provides a wealth of resources to help you learn how to create models. The best way to learn how to create a neural network is to follow along with some of the excellent YouTube videos. Josh Starmer's Neural Networks videos are a good general introduction. https://www.youtube.com/watch?v=CqOfi41LfDw&list=PLblh5JKOoLUIxGDQs4LFFD--41Vzf-ME1.

For specific information on how to code a neural network in R, view this Liquid Brain video:

https://www.youtube.com/watch?v=RKJfZPNYCsA.

Chapter 19 also provides a wealth of resources to help you learn how to create models.

Backpropagation is a method that neural networks use to learn how to improve. The difference between what the model predicts and the truth is a measure of wrongness. For example, suppose the patient had cancer but the model predicted a probability of cancer of 0.85, the error would be 0.15 ($1.0-0.85 = 0.15$). This might be referred to as a residual or a loss. With many iterations, the neural network algorithm reweights the predictors to minimize this degree of wrongness, in reverse order. For more information about backpropagation, see Josh Starmer's video: https://www.youtube.com/watch?v=CqOfi41LfDw&list=PLblh5JKOoLUIxGDQs4LFFD--41Vzf-ME1.

Deep learning is a neural network with many layers. Each layer can capture some aspect of the variables inputted to improve the prediction.

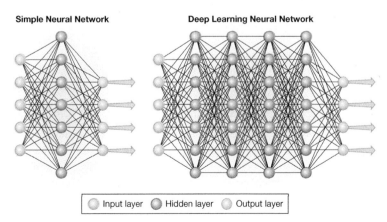

FIGURE 6.2. Neural networks and deep learning. Neural networks take input predictors and convert them to outputs by iteratively weighting the values. Deep learning is an extension of a neural network that can have many hidden layers, which provide for the transformation and extraction of features for much more advanced models.

ML has many strengths and will be used to improve many aspects of medicine, but there have been problems that need to be addressed. Many of the evaluations have been weak, biased, or nonexistent. Much of the reporting has not included a balanced account of the pros and cons of various approaches.

ML became more popular than traditional statistical approaches for a number of reasons. Primarily, the ML approach will always supply an answer, while with traditional statistical approaches the answer sometimes is: "We cannot make an accurate prediction."

Some criticize deep learning as simply neural networks rebranded and that there is nothing new. These critics will claim that this technology is 25 years old and because it was proven to be a failure before, it has been rebranded as something new, that is "deep learning." This is untrue. Major advances have been made to enable the success of modern deep learning tools, such faster computers, more powerful chips, and many more hidden layers in the network. In addition, the following specific forms of deep learning have provided remarkable success stories.

Convolutional Neural Networks (CNNs) or "ConvNet"—a type of deep learning algorithm often used in imaging analyses with spatial structure to slide patches, or kernels, over an image. CNNs use these moving grids across an image to pass information to a local neighbor, thus creating models that learn about the structure. A regular neural network uses a general matrix multiplication. Convolutional networks are a specialized type of neural networks that use convolution in place of general matrix multiplication in at least one of their layers. CNNs were a major advance used by DeepMind to predict protein structures in AlphaFold. To learn more about CNNs, watch the following video by Sander Dieleman: "DeepMind x UCL Lecture 3, Deep Learning Lectures, Convolutional Neural Networks for Image Recognition." https://www.youtube.com/watch?v=shVKhOmT0HE.

Recurrent Neural Networks (RNNs)—can handle a sequence of inputs, such as patient laboratory data on day 1, day 2, day 3, etc. Standard feedforward neural networks cannot handle this type of data. With RNNs, data are ordered in a sequence and information flows sequentially. A RETAIN-based model is an advanced variation of an RNN. RETAIN: an interpretable predictive model for health care using REverse Time AttentIoN mechanism. https://arxiv.org/abs/1608.05745. Long short-term memory is a technique used in artificial recurrent neural networks for deep learning. This provides a method of moving from a single data point to a sequence of data.

Generative Adversarial Networks—Two neural networks generate new data sets and then compete with one another. For example, one (generator) creates CT images with cancer and the other (discriminator) tries to detect the fakes. The generator creates fake data and the discriminator tests to learn fake data from real data.

Decision trees

Decision Tree is a tree-like flowchart model that splits on the most important predictor and continues to the next most important predictor (Figure 6.3). Decision trees are computationally intensive algorithms that try to minimize

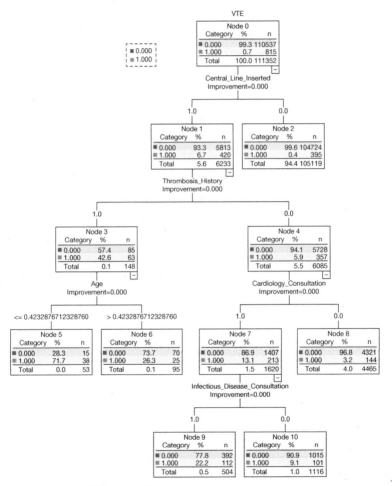

FIGURE 6.3. CART—Classification and regression tree. In this decision tree, one can see that the overall rate of venous thromboembolism (VTE) is 0.7% in the top node. The predictor variable of "central line inserted" is coded as 1 = yes and 0 = no. Those with a central line have a VTE rate of 6.7%, while those without a central line have a rate of 0.4%. The model continues to divide based on the next most important predictor.

the impurity by selecting the optimal predictors and optimal cut points. The advantages of decision trees include that they are explainable and easy to create. The disadvantages include that a large data set is required to create a robust model and the information is dichotomized and not used in an optimal fashion.

Random Forest—is an ensemble learning method that works by creating many decision trees and then combining them. A disadvantage of using this technique is that the model needs many events (outcomes) per predictor variable. The models generally perform better than decision trees but not as well as gradient boosted trees.

Gradient boosted decision trees—an ML technique that uses an ensemble of decisions trees to optimize prediction through successive steps.

XGBoost—XGBoost is a package of powerful ML tools that has gained popularity because it was used by teams who won several modeling competitions. Although these techniques are powerful, they can result in overfitting and users need to be alert for reverse causation. For Python users, scikit-learn can run XGBoost and for R users the caret package will do this.

---

i FOR MORE INFORMATION

StatQuest. Neural Networks Pt. 1: Inside the Black Box. Josh Starmer.[9]

MIT "Introduction to Deep Learning". Foundations of Deep Learning. Alexander Amini.[10]

AlphaGo. The Movie | Full award-winning documentary. Greg Kohs (director).[11]

Reinforcement Learning online course (13 lectures) by Hado van Hasselt. DeepMind × UCL.

https://www.youtube.com/watch?v=TCCjZe0y4Qc.

Reinforcement Learning: An Introduction. By Richard S. Sutton and Andrew G. Barto

http://incompleteideas.net/book/the-book-2nd.html

http://incompleteideas.net/book/RLbook2020.pdf.

Population median imputation was noninferior to complex approaches for imputing missing values in cardiovascular prediction models in clinical practice. By Gijs Berkelmans et al.[12]

CHAPTER SUMMARY

Devote the time to select an AI project that is likely to succeed and then develop a playbook as the strategic plan. Keep an open mind about potential predictors and start with a comprehensive data dictionary. Study the TRIPOD guidelines to ensure your approach is modern and robust and will enable you to publish your paper in a high-profile journal. Be agnostic about the modeling technique, try several and use the method that provides the best results. Understand the strengths and weaknesses of the various approaches and be completely transparent about both. Be open-minded about predictor variables but avoid the common errors of circular logic and overfitting. Have a strategic plan which includes the Domenico Guidelines and adapt the model after consideration of the tactics available.

REFERENCES

1. Mühlenbruch K, Jeppesen C, Joost HG, Boeing H, Schulze MB. The value of genetic information for diabetes risk prediction—differences according to sex, age, family history and obesity. *PLoS One.* 2013;8(5):e64307. Erratum in: *PLoS One.* 2013;8(9).
2. Warner JL, Zhang P, Liu J, Alterovitz G. Classification of hospital acquired complications using temporal clinical information from a large electronic health record. *J Biomed Inf.* 2016;59:209-217.
3. Walker SC, Creech CB, Domenico HJ, French B, Byrne DW, Wheeler AP. A real-time risk-prediction model for pediatric venous thromboembolic events. *Pediatrics.* 2021;147(6):e2020042325.
4. Riley RD, Ensor J, Snell KIE, et al. Calculating the sample size required for developing a clinical prediction model. *BMJ.* 2020;368:m441.
5. Byrne D. *Publishing Your Medical Research.* Wolters Kluwer; 2017. https://www.slideshare.net/DanielByrne12/publishing-your-medical-research-125452257
6. Chen JH, Altman RB. Data-mining electronic medical records for clinical order recommendations: wisdom of the crowd or tyranny of the mob? *AMIA Jt Summits Transl Sci Proc.* 2015;2015:435-439. Accessed September 20, 2022. https://www.ncbi.nlm.nih.gov/pmc/articles/PMC4525236/
7. Choi PJ, Curlin FA, Cox CE. "The patient is dying, please call the chaplain": the activities of chaplains in one medical center's intensive care units. *J Pain Symptom Manag.* 2015;50:501-506.

8. Zuo L, Du X, Zhao W, et al. Improving anticoagulant treatment strategies of atrial fibrillation using reinforcement learning. *AMIA Annu Symp Proc.* 2021;2020:1431-1440.

9. Starmer J. StatQuest. Neural Networks Pt. 1: Inside the Black Box. https://www.youtube.com/watch?v=CqOfi41LfDw

10. Amini A. Foundations of deep learning. https://www.youtube.com/watch?v=WXuK6gekU1Y. MIT "Introduction to Deep Learning"

11. AlphaGo. The Movie | Full award-winning documentary. Greg Kohs (director). https://www.youtube.com/watch?v=WXuK6gekU1Y

12. Berkelmans GFN, Read SH, Gudbjörnsdottir S, et al. Population median imputation was noninferior to complex approaches for imputing missing values in cardiovascular prediction models in clinical practice. *J Clin Epidemiol.* 2022;145:70-80. doi:10.1016/j.jclinepi.2022.01.011. PMID: 35066115.

7

EHRs—Exporting, Cleaning, Managing Datasets, and Integrating Models into the Electronic Health Record

> *"There is no AI without IA—Information Architecture."*
> —Seth Early.

PRINCIPLE 69 • **The EHR systems were designed to improve hospital billing not to be data sources for research or AI.**

Electronic health record (EHR) information is plentiful, but health care leaders must prepare for the future by investing in resources to build a strong information architecture to ensure data reliability, completeness, and useability.

Information Architecture (IA) refers to a system for storing, structuring, organizing, and labeling data in a format that can be easily used. Interoperability is the ability of computer systems or software to exchange and make use of information. For example, most statistical software packages require that the data be structured and coded in one flat file—a spreadsheet—with variables names in the top row and the first patient's data in the second row with a separate column for each variable. The EHR was not designed with this in mind. From an organizational standpoint, there were problems in the EHR data that did not matter for billing—but do now for Artificial Intelligence (AI) projects. For example, the percent of patients with data on body mass index, smoking status, and exercise level should be tracked over time and improved as a continuous quality improvement project to gradually improve the usefulness of the data.

Exporting data from the EHR is a common bottleneck in building AI tools

Most of the current EHRs record raw unstructured data but fail to combine the information to make it more useful and predictive. This would be analogous to a weather person on TV who simply reports the current local temperature and wind speed but does not combine any of the information into weather models. By combining large amounts of structured, coded weather data in models, the weather person can provide accurate and precise forecast predictions. This is the value that they provide and the next step for health care.

PRINCIPLE 70 • Data is the new oil, but like oil, it needs to be processed before it is useful.

Data management is an important part of the process of transforming EHR data into a useful AI tool. Successful health care organizations recognize the need for this specialty and are investing in recruiting and paying talented experts in this area. These informatics experts are skilled at merging files, recoding text into codes, and handling missing data in a sophisticated way.

Successful health care organizations will quickly and efficiently export data, build models, and add them into the EHR

It is technically possible to (1) export a data set needed to create a predictive model from the EHR in 1 day, (2) create an excellent predictive model in 1 day, and (3) code the model into the EHR in 1 day. Most models can be tested in a pragmatic randomized controlled trial in about 1 year. But this process can take forever. To fix this, forward-thinking health care leaders will decide that this is a priority and put resources into it. They will hire skilled, experience people to be on the AI development team. These people will not try to accomplish this work in their spare time when they have no other demands on them but will be devoted to these projects. The leaders will be very hands-on to move these projects along and help overcome obstacle.

Natural language processing (NLP) can convert dictation into EHR progress notes. These tools must be assessed with randomization to ensure that they actually do improve accuracy and clinician satisfaction.

AI speech recognition tools can convert dictated progress notes into text. Physicians then edit this version and submit rather than starting from scratch. The impact of this change needs to be studied with rigor. Recent research has shown that some of these tools that appear to solve problems actually cause problems and increase the workload.[1]

NLP is progressing and assisting with unstructured data in the EHR; however, much work remains to be done.

NLP refers to AI tools that process written or spoken language. Although there is much discussion about the unstructured text data in the EHR and the need for NLP to use these data for AI, the structured data (age, sex, laboratory data, ICD codes) work well and are a feasible option for many AI models today. NLP has value and will grow as the methods become more sophisticated.

The AI work on NLP is nothing magical. Much of it has to do with searching for key words, such as "lupus" and identifying negation of the term "rule out lupus." Machine learning can be used to identify other patterns that help refine the match. Much of the NLP work could be avoided by entering more health care data in a structured way rather than allowing extensive free text and subsequent clean up.

Rather than recording most of the data as free text and subsequently developing NLP tools to extract small percentages of the information, EHRs should evolve to record more information with structured formatting.

For example, rather than a text sentence about smoking history, it should be recorded in a structured way (Figure 7.1) such as follows:

1. Is this patient a current cigarette smoker? 0—no, 1—yes.
2. If yes, number of packs per day.
3. If yes, number of years smoking.
4. If no, is this patient a former smoker? 0—no, 1—yes.
5. If a former smoker, years since quitting.

This type of data entry is no more difficult or time consuming and improves the completeness and usefulness of the data. The current data entry approach is broken, and incentives need to be created to modify intake forms and change data entry behavior.

case	smoker	packs_per_day	yrs_smoking	former_smoker	yrs_since_quit	pack_yrs	smoking history (unstructured text)
1	1	2	15	0	0	30	Patient reports a history of smoking
2	0	0	0	0	0	0	(blank)
3	0	0	0	0	0	0	nonsmoker
4	1	1	40	0	0	40	History of tobacco use

FIGURE 7.1. An example of structured and unstructured data. With structured data, the variables are stored in a consistent manner and often coded, allowing for use in AI projects. Unstructured data are free form text, string variables, which require natural language processing. These variables are more challenging to use in AI models.

PRINCIPLE 71 • Capture information in the health records that is linked to patient-centered short-term and long-term health outcomes.

"If you cannot measure it, you cannot improve it."

— Lord Kelvin.

One of the major shortcomings of the current EHRs is a lack of short-term and long-term outcomes data. Record outcomes that are important to the patient, not simply a process metric or what is important to the physician or hospital (Table 7.1). For example, a hospital may consider patient care a success if they are discharged alive, but the solution is to measure success from the patient's perspective, as Wes Ely, M.D., pointed out in his excellent book, *"Every Deep-Drawn Breath: A Critical Care Doctor on Healing, Recovery, and Transforming Medicine in the ICU."*[2] Much of the time, doctors have limited data about whether their decisions led to improvements for their patient. This feedback loop is essential.

If we do not measure the things that matter most, such as the overall long-term health, then we risk an overemphasis on short-term metrics that are poor proxies for what we really care about. A system with only short-term

TABLE 7.1	Important Patient-Centric Outcome Variables That Should be Routinely Collected

Survival (survived/died, date of death, or date of last follow-up)

Hospital readmission (this is often missing for readmissions to other hospitals)

Activities of daily living

Quality of life

Days to return to prehospital status (work or school)

Functional status

Level of pain

Patient satisfaction

Quality-Adjusted Life Year (QALY)—these range from 1 (perfect health) to 0 (dead). One year in perfect health is equal to 1 QALY.

Patient Reported Outcome Measures—quality measures derived from patient reported information.

Overall health score (0 = dead to 100 = optimal health)

metrics can result in AI tools which simply optimize surrogate end points. Many AI projects require the development of new robust metrics which capture and manage information with linkage to long-term outcomes databases. This is especially true for AI studies such as screening mammograms.

Decentralized health care data are a problem that makes it challenging to build medical AI tools. Medical information is stored in multiple locations for a given patient, but the short-term and long-term health outcomes are often not recorded—or stored in completely different computer system. One solution is to have a unique identifier for each person so that it is possible to merge data sets. A national patient identifier, or ID number, would enable long-term health outcome information to be used in smarter ways, which would help with forward progress of AI evaluations. Common data elements standards are needed for advancing AI in medicine. Progress in medical AI requires standards for how variables are named and how values are recorded.

The culture in biomedical informatics has historically avoided randomization, but this is changing. Successful biomedical informatics leaders have realized that many of the informatics tools embedded in the EHR are easy to randomize and the results are crucial to forward progress. This change in culture will be important in mobilizing these talented experts to solve the important problems that have held medical AI back.

> *"We believe there is an urgent need to promote the use of RCTs of clinical information systems, given continuing reservations in the medical informatics community."*
>
> —JOSEPH LIU AND JEREMY WYATT.[3]

> *"The RCT is an important and powerful method, and an underused one in medical informatics."*
>
> —JOSEPH LIU.[3,4]

PRINCIPLE 72 • Creating one general AI predictive model for a health condition or medical complication across the entire hospital is often possible and preferable.

The assumption that each department or specialty would require a different model is often false. In our work building predictive models of hospital complications, one overall model performed as well as the models designed for a subgroup of patients. For most conditions, it is not feasible to create a model for each department or unit in the hospital when one model could be used for the entire adult hospital. The work that would be required to code and maintain multiple models in the EHR for the same condition would not be worth the effort. Separate models will, however, be needed for certain situations, such as the children's hospital. If a group insists on a specific model for their own unit, they must demonstrate why this additional expense is justified. In general, a variable can be added to a model, such as trauma, rather than creating another model for trauma patients.

For example, the Braden Scale is used across hospitals for pressure injury risk assessment. There is not a different version for each department. There is not a different Braden Scale on days 2, 3, 4, etc, for the patients' stay. Many of the specialty-specific models were driven more by the desire to publish a paper rather than the need.

A successful health care organization will build on an existing predictive model by incorporating predictors and interactions to make it more accurate for the various clinical departments—model 101, model 102, etc. This approach is also better for grantsmanship and publishing papers in high-profile journals.

PRINCIPLE 73 • For implementation to be successful, use the continuous probability of outcome and avoid dichotomizing risk.

Display the continuous probability of an AI predictive model and do not simplify to a dichotomized alert as high/low, or an ordinal alert—green/yellow/red. A surprising number of predictive models and scoring systems commit the double sin of dichotomizing twice. They will dichotomize the input predictors (BMI = obese) and dichotomize the output probability (high risk for blood clot). This is an unnecessary waste of valuable information.

The models provide a probability of the outcome. These can be color-coded to also provide categories for implementation (low, medium, high risk), but the probabilities should always be displayed, thereby providing information needed for risk stratification. Defining the categories can be performed as part of the implementation. Implementation should not be delayed in order to define categories.

In one system, risk of patients falling in the hospital was color-coded. All of the patients on a unit in the hospital had a red alert icon next to their name, meaning they were high risk. Therefore, the nurses ignored the alert. If all patients are high risk, it defeats the purpose of risk stratification. It is always better to show the granularity of risk. The color coding can also be used, but an effective system includes the probability of the outcome.

To look at the Braden Scale again, most hospitals currently use the Braden Scale and then dichotomize the patients in the hospital as high or low risk for pressure injury. This approach is flawed because too many patients are lumped into high risk, the system fails to include other factors that predict pressure injury, and it fails to use the power of computers in assessing risk with finer granularity (Figure 7.2).

Accurate, automated, and timely risk stratification is needed to improve most measurements in health care. The high-risk patients need certain prevention resources and the low-risk patients do not.

Variables in the Equation

		B	S.E.	Wald	df	Sig.	Exp(B)	95% C.I.for EXP(B) Lower	Upper
Step 1[a]	Central_Line_Inserted(1)	1.583	.093	287.507	1	<.001	4.870	4.056	5.849
	Thrombosis_History(1)	2.156	.137	246.884	1	<.001	8.639	6.602	11.305
	Cardiology_Consultation (1)	1.436	.093	238.433	1	<.001	4.205	3.504	5.045
	Blood_Gases_Measured (1)	1.121	.096	137.371	1	<.001	3.068	2.544	3.700
	Infectious_Disease_Con sultation(1)	.932	.088	111.263	1	<.001	2.539	2.135	3.019
	Age	.056	.006	85.209	1	<.001	1.058	1.045	1.070
	MCHC	−.147	.029	26.313	1	<.001	.863	.816	.913
	CANCER(1)	.486	.111	19.173	1	<.001	1.625	1.308	2.020
	RDW	.059	.017	11.603	1	<.001	1.061	1.025	1.098
	Lactate	.079	.029	7.208	1	.007	1.082	1.022	1.146
	Surgical_Procedure(1)	.045	.117	.146	1	.703	1.046	.831	1.315
	Constant	−2.537	1.117	5.159	1	.023	.079		

a. Variable(s) entered on step 1: Central_Line_Inserted, Thrombosis_History, Cardiology_Consultation, Blood_Gases _Measured, Infectious_Disease _Consultation, Age, MCHC, CANCER, RDW, Lactate, Surgical_Procedure.

FIGURE 7.2. Converting statistical output into a useable formula. Statistical software packages will display output similar to this for a logistic regression model. The intercept is listed as a constant here. Each variable in the model has a weight or beta coefficient listed under B. To compute the probability of a venous thromboembolism (VTE) for a given patient, one would multiply the patient's values by the coefficients. For example, age would be multiplied by 0.056. The probability of a VTE would be $1/(1+ [2.7183]$ ^$(-Z)) \times 100$. Round to one decimal place and display as a percent. Where $Z = -2.537 + (2.156 \times 1$ if patient has a history of thrombosis, 0 otherwise) + (0.045 × 1 if surgical procedure performed during this encounter, 0 otherwise) + (0.486 × 1 if patient has a diagnosis of cancer, 0 otherwise) + (0.932 × 1 if infectious disease consult ordered this encounter, 0 otherwise) + (1.436 × 1 if cardiology consult ordered this encounter, 0 otherwise) + (1.121 × 1 if blood gas lab panel was ordered this encounter, 0 otherwise) + (1.583 × 1 if patient has a central line present, 0 otherwise) + (0.056 × patient age in years) + (−0.147 × patient mean corpuscular hemoglobin concentration (MCHC). If MCHC is missing, impute a value of 34.0) + (0.059 × patient red cell distribution width (RDW). If RDW is missing, impute a value of 14.3) + (0.079 × patient lactate. If lactate is missing, impute a value of 1.3).

These limited resources are often provided to patients without accurate risk stratification, which means that many of the high-risk patients do not receive the prevention that they need (Figure 1.5). In one project, researchers found that among the patients with the highest risk of a pressure injury, the known prevention was only performed about 50% of the time. So, the AI model works by checking and rechecking that the known prevention checklist is performed for the highest risk patients in a timely and reliable way.

PRINCIPLE 74 • Enable users to notify the model developer/researchers of errors, and use this to adapt and improve the model.

Adding a mechanism which would allow the user to send feedback such as "This does not look right" is a way to build in a feedback loop and to continuously improve and correct faulty models. Feedback might be as vague as "The model says X but I think it should be Y." This can also be used to flag a potential bias that should be investigated.

Additionally, develop a feedback loop for understanding when and why the clinician ignores the AI recommendation. This is an important part of the implementation research, and can be collected by the centralized implementation person, or as a part of the alert. The alert can prompt the user to provide a justification for ignoring the recommendation.

The effectiveness of AI-related interventions must be assessed with feedback loops, which often do not exist and need to be developed for the evaluation.

Reasoning needs to be collected from those who ignore evidence-based recommendation alerts. The implementation work needs to account for clinical situations in which it was appropriate to ignore. For the others, there needs to be an appropriate nudge or escalation.

Use augmented vigilance with automatic escalation in a closed loop system to be more effective than the average alert.

If clinicians ignore the alert, there will be an appropriate escalation. The goal is to improve end-to-end performance.

If the clinician changes a behavior based on the alert, there is no escalation, but if not, the next level up alert is prompted. This process continues until the intervention is performed or until there is a valid reason documented for not doing so. For example, a car's seat belt alert uses a form of escalation which moves from a red icon to a beeping sound to an annoying and continuous alarm. Implementation research is extremely important and often given inadequate attention.

PRINCIPLE 75 • After AI tools are implemented, have a post-deployment surveillance to assess for performance drift.

Periodically, assessment of the model's performance should be made by a standing data and safety monitoring board with an auditing of the inputs and outputs for a random sample of patients. Remember, you are chasing a moving target and models need to be revalidated periodically to ensure that they still perform as expected. Here calibration drift detection systems can be useful for deciding when to update the model.[5]

PRINCIPLE 76 • Ironically, the goal is to break the AI model. The goal is to prevent a complication in the patient predicted to have one. In this way, the outcome will change in the intervention group compared with the control group.

Ironically, the long-term goal of a predictive model project is to have the model become obsolete! The implementation team is constantly trying to prove that the model is wrong. If the model successfully predicts when patients will develop a condition or complication, and the hospital resources are focused on preventing that high-risk patient from developing that complication, then prospectively, the model will appear to no longer predict as well as before or as expected. Of course, this will not happen in the control group and therefore we can assess cause-effect during the trial.

PRINCIPLE 77 • Build models that are robust to dataset shifts. Brittle models are a major problem in AI.

Brittleness is the tendency of a model to be easily fooled with slight changes in the data. This is the opposite of robustness and stability. Brittleness causes the model to fail to generalize in other settings for a variety of reasons: different equipment, different practice patterns, different names for predictors, etc.

Dataset shift refers to the fact that within a health care system and EHR the model that was built on data from years ago may not perform appropriately today.[6,7] The solution to this problem is to reassess the model periodically. Is the rate of the outcome similar today as when the model was built? Are these predictors still the most important factors?

Building robust and fair models requires evaluations to address accidental fitting of confounders, unintended discriminatory bias, the challenges of generalization to new populations, and the unintended negative consequences of new algorithms on health outcomes.[4]

PRINCIPLE 78 • Get data on the person—not just the patient.

Health care systems that record a comprehensive set of predictors and execute structured health risk assessments (HRAs) annually will have the data needed to create and use modern AI tools (Figure 7.3). They will have the data they need to intervene, thereby changing the outcomes. This will give them the competitive advantage over other hospitals. One method to obtain additional structured data is to ask patients to complete an annual HRA

Health Condition	Currently diagnosed			Probability	
		Undiagnosed	1 Year	5 Years	10 Years
Diabetes	100%				
Hypercholesteremia	100%				
Hemochromatosis		92%	92%	92%	92%
Hypertension		87%	90%	90%	90%
Multiple myeloma		50%	55%	60%	65%
Mental health condition		4%	5%	6%	6%
Prostate cancer		2%	3%	4%	4%
Melanoma skin cancer		2%	3%	3%	3%
Chronic liver disease/cirrhosis		2%	2%	3%	4%
COVID-19		2%	1%	0%	0%
Heart disease		1%	3%	10%	12%
Cancer		1%	3%	5%	10%
Heart attack		1%	2%	3%	3%
Influenza/pneumonia		1%	2%	2%	2%
Lung cancer		1%	2%	2%	2%
Stroke/cerebrovascular disease		1%	1%	2%	4%
Kidney disease		1%	1%	2%	2%
Parkinson disease		1%	1%	2%	2%
Alzheimer disease		1%	1%	1%	2%
Chronic lung disease		1%	1%	1%	1%
Blood infection		1%	1%	1%	1%
Suicidal ideation		1%	1%	1%	1%
Congestive heart failure		1%	1%	1%	1%
Colorectal cancer		1%	1%	1%	1%
Autoimmune disease		1%	1%	1%	1%
Lupus		1%	1%	1%	1%
Gastric cancer		1%	1%	1%	1%
Obesity		0%	2%	2%	2%
Atrial fibrillation		0%	0%	0%	1%
Breast cancer		0%	0%	0%	0%
Cervical cancer		0%	0%	0%	0%
Ovarian cancer		0%	0%	0%	0%

FIGURE 7.3. Vaporware of what a primary care provider will see in the EHR at an annual checkup. Vaporware is software that is a concept and has not been completely developed. In the future, physicians will have tools like this available to them to decrease the burden of information overload. Each probability will be based on a predictive model converting the patients' values into outputs.

form. Another option for building a data set that could help improve patient outcomes is to periodically survey patients with validated measurement tools. Or use the 23andMe method of periodically emailing a few specific questions, such as "How often do you consciously choose to eat more fiber in your meals or snacks?" or "In a typical week, do you regularly take any vitamin or mineral supplements?" This method is a way to collect structured data that patients voluntarily contribute.

Patients should be offered an incentive to complete an HRA when they are new patients in the system, and then annually. This will provide structured data that can be used to predict outcome and intervention that can improve their health. Most EHRs are filled with information about illness, but the HRA collects information about diet, exercise, stress, and lifestyle. All of this work, of course, must be performed with complete transparency and the highest ethical standards. Many patients are altruistic and willing to contribute to projects that can help them or someone else.

Physicians and nurses waste huge amounts of time interviewing new patients and typing their information into the EHR. Most of this could be performed by patients online before their first visit. AI can help streamline the documentation, but it requires redesigning the workflow. Web sites and applications like MyChart are the perfect place to collect this HRA information.

Clinicians sometimes dismiss self-reported data from an HRA as being less reliable than the EHR data. This is a complex topic, but much of the self-reported data in an HRA are much more reliable, complete, and feasible to work with than the data in the EHR. In many ways, this is a smarter alternative than creating a massive amount of unstructured data and then developing AI NLP tools to try to fix it. A successful approach would be more like TurboTax. TurboTax does not allow you to enter paragraphs of free text about your finances and tax situation for the past year and then try to apply NLP to fix it. Instead, the software will ask you specific questions with branching logic to collect answers that are useable. The data are structured enabling the software to provide value by saving the user time in completing their taxes. The results are highly reliable because there is no noise from an NLP text conversion. Present systems could convert the important parts of free text in the EHR to something similar to TurboTax. There will always be a need to enter free text, but it must be gradually reduced, and the structured data must be gradually but significantly increased.

When collecting structured data, some are concerned about violating copyright laws if the questions are part of a "copyrighted" inventory or scoring system. Few people realize this, but forms designed to collect data are not covered under the U.S. copyright protection. "Blank forms that are designed for recording information and do not themselves convey information are uncopyrightable." This is important in health care AI work so that data can be collected in a uniform and reproducible manner. You can use the same wording as is used in a survey.

ℹ️ FOR MORE INFORMATION

Cleveland Clinic Risk Calculator Library. Michael Kattan.[8]
Works Not Protected by Copyright. U.S. Copyright Office · Library of Congress
https://www.copyright.gov/circs/circ33.pdf.

CHAPTER SUMMARY

As hospitals increasingly rely on EHRs for not only billing but also research and real-time AI tools, more effort needs to be devoted to continuously improving the completeness and accuracy of the data in the EHR—the IA. Common data elements—standardized key terms—have been discussed for decades, but strong leadership and funding is needed for more progress in this area. NLP can help with some problems but at the same time more of the medical information needs to be stored in a useable, structured, and coded format. Long-term, patient-centric measures are needed to create AI tools that matter. Leadership must enable teams to build and improve upon previous models. The wasted resources of creating hundreds of unused models must be focused on building model 102, 103, to keep improving on existing overall models. Oversight from health care leaders is needed to guide the portfolio of AI work to building on previous successes and moving forward. Without this, researchers will continue to create models that are never implemented.

REFERENCES

1. Payne TH, Alonso WD, Markiel JA, et al. Using voice to create inpatient progress notes: effects on note timeliness, quality, and physician satisfaction. *JAMIA Open*. 2018;1(2):218-226.
2. Ely W. *Every Deep-Drawn Breath: A Critical Care Doctor on Healing, Recovery, and Transforming Medicine in the ICU.* Scribner; 2021.
3. Liu JL, Wyatt JC. The case for randomized controlled trials to assess the impact of clinical information systems. *J Am Med Inform Assoc*. 2011;18(2):173-180.

4. Liu JL, Wyatt JC, Deeks JJ, et al. Systematic reviews of clinical decision tools for acute abdominal pain. *Health Technol Assess.* 2006;10(47):1-167, iii-iv.

5. Davis SE, Greevy RA, Jr, Lasko TA, Walsh CG, Matheny ME. Detection of calibration drift in clinical prediction models to inform model updating. *J Biomed Inform.* 2020;112:103611.

6. Nestor B, McDermott MBA, Chauhan G, et al. Rethinking clinical prediction: why machine learning must consider year of care and feature aggregation. In: Machine Learning for Health (ML4H).

7. Davis SE, Greevy RA, Fonnesbeck C, Lasko TA, Walsh CG, Matheny ME. A nonparametric updating method to correct clinical prediction model drift. *J Am Med Inform Assoc.* 2019;26(12):1448-1457.

8. Kattan M. Cleveland clinic risk calculator library. http://riskcalc.org:3838/

The Implementation

Resistance—Understanding and Overcoming the Resistance to AI, Randomization, and Change

> *"The measure of intelligence is the ability to change."*
> —ALBERT EINSTEIN.

Making intelligent decisions often requires balancing the probability of benefit with the probability of harm or risk. The antiscience, data-free arguments of those who refuse the COVID-19 vaccine illustrate how many people are unable to balance these. This inability to make balanced decisions often results in irrational excuses that slow the AI process. The first step in overcoming the resistance to Artificial Intelligence (AI), randomization, and change in general is to try to understand it.

> *"The amount of energy needed to refute bullshit is an order of magnitude larger than is needed to produce it."*
> —BRANDOLINI'S LAW, ALSO KNOWN AS THE BULLSHIT ASYMMETRY PRINCIPLE.[1-3]

In our current health care system, some have a myopic view similar to taxi drivers in 2009—before Uber. Their attitude was "We have a monopoly and can charge what we want and provide the quality of service that we want."

The resistance to AI in medicine is similar to the concerns people have about all new technology—electricity, telephone, cars, the PC—but nearly all of the predicted fiascos of late have been false, or society found a way to prevent or circumvent the problem. Biostatisticians will need to be at the frontline of these changes. In the past, some would criticize AI and become obstacles to forward progress. Although some of their criticism was valid, biostatisticians need to not only become involved in the implementation of AI, but they need to become leaders at building and rigorously testing the impact on health outcomes. Their expertise in model development, evaluations, and randomized controlled trials is needed to move AI to the next level.

> *"I could not bring myself to believe that if knowledge presented danger, the solution was ignorance. To me, it always seemed that the solution had to be wisdom. You did not refuse to look at danger, rather you learned how to handle it safely."*
>
> —Isaac Asimov.

PRINCIPLE 79 • Health care leaders need to start with a common goal, articulate a long-term vision to rally the organization, and make it clear that "Health care is AI-ready, and the status quo is dead!"

Health care leaders of high-performance organizations will send a positive message, "We are going to win on innovation!" Health care managers must be catalysts to improve the rate of forward progress, to challenge the status quo, and support evidence-based technology. This will require education and restructuring of the organization to support assessing AI with rigor. Although they do not need to perform the technical AI coding work, senior leaders do need to stay involved with the AI projects and solve implementation problems.

As a developer, demonstrate that the best way to achieve the common goal is with scientific rigor. Communicate and educate until you have support from leadership, faculty, the Institutional Review Board, and hospital operations staff. Align an AI project with the hospital's overall goals so it is not seen as a hindrance to what is important.

A sometimes-overlooked aspect of what health care leaders must communicate is that this is a great place to work. Yet, gaming the system with flawed evaluations results in burnout and turnover. People want to be part of something new and exciting. Morale and retention improve when an institution successfully improves health outcomes with modern science and technology.

> *"We live in a world where unfortunately the distinction between true and false appears to become increasingly blurred by manipulation of facts, by exploitation of uncritical minds, and by the pollution of the language."*
>
> —Arne Tiselius, Swedish biochemist and 1948 Nobel Laureate.

PRINCIPLE 80 • Avoid stepped wedge designs like the plague, especially if it is possible to use patient-level randomization for testing AI.

"I write because there is some lie that I want to expose, some fact to which I want to draw attention."

—GEORGE ORWELL.

Rather than truly randomize, some will use a stepped wedge design, but the stepped wedge trial design is a very weak type of randomized controlled trial. In a patient-level randomized controlled trial, participants are randomly assigned individually to either the control group or the treatment group. In some clinical settings, this is difficult or impossible. The stepped wedge provides a design in which participants can be assigned to the treatment arm in waves or steps.

All patients are in the control group at the beginning and then clusters are moved into the treatment arm; thus, the study design diagram looks like steps. The clusters may be units in a hospital or hospitals in a network.

Stepped wedge designs should be avoided as they are inefficient and rarely lead to success. Theoretically, the stepped wedge design is a good option. In practice, it often leads to failure due to several challenges. Few researchers have the resources or authority to conduct the stepped wedge in a rigorous way. It requires enormous resources for collecting data in every cluster before and during the entire trial. Second, the design is only valid if the units are started in a random order. Many researchers are unable to accomplish this and many start in the unit or hospital with the largest problem—the outlier. This results in regression to the mean and a conclusion "proving" that the intervention worked. Third, during the study period, it is highly likely that there will be changes in health care that impact the outcome, which can be challenging to untangle from the intervention. Fourth, the analysis of the data is much more complex to conduct and communicate.

Although many fans of stepped wedge studies enthusiastically promote the advantages, the results are very disappointing. Often groups will start a stepped wedge and begin in the unit of the hospital that has the largest problem, realize how challenging the full study will be, and then convert the stepped wedge into a before-after study in one unit. Regression to the mean again guarantees that this outlier moves closer to baseline, which results in pseudo-success. These papers often get published in very low-impact journals where the peer review process is weak. Only 2 of 47,476 papers in *The New England Journal of Medicine* used a stepped wedge study design. If this was a strong study design, it would be used by more than 0.004% of researchers who are publishing in this top journal. If it is possible to randomize at the patient level, do so. If not, consider a cluster-crossover, but first study the challenges. For studies of AI in medicine, avoid stepped wedge designs at all costs.

"It is not necessary to change. Survival is not mandatory."
—W. E. DEMING.

PRINCIPLE 81 • **Some will say that to successfully implement and test AI in medicine you need to involve physicians. This is the wrong approach. Physicians must lead the project—not just be involved. For nursing projects, nurses must lead.**

Although engineers, computer scientists, AI experts, and biostatisticians are very smart, they often fail to understand how decisions are made in a hospital and how health care workflows function. So, approach implementation of AI in medicine with a new and sophisticated level of understanding to avoid future resistance. Empowering physician-scientists will "democratize" data and analytics to enable them to derive value from AI.

By eliciting their input in creating the data dictionary of potential predictors, this becomes their model—not a model imposed on them. This team involvement will dramatically increase the odds of adoption. The key is to involve the clinical team from the beginning in all aspects of the model development, testing, implementation, and publication. You must build an AI team and continuously improve it to get the right people on and the wrong people off the team. The ultimate goal is to earn the trust of clinicians and give them the gift of time so that they can do what they love—spend more time with patients.

Although it is possible to use end-to-end machine learning to automatically create complex machine learning models and exclude physicians and biostatisticians, the results often suffer. Many of the previous applications of AI in medicine were failures of teamwork not technology. The failed approach was caused by AI people talking briefly with domain experts—"I talked with a doc in the hospital and he said X." This is the wrong approach.

PRINCIPLE 82 • **Document the need for clinical decision support by demonstrating that clinicians are not reliably predicting, classifying, and agreeing with one another. Ideally, have one of the clinical team members do this from the inside.**

"The difficulty lies not so much in developing new ideas as in escaping from old ones."
—JOHN MAYNARD KEYNES.

One obstacle is that some clinicians believe that they do not need AI. They can already identify which patients will be readmitted, develop a blood clot, or have a pressure injury. Some radiologists believe that they can detect breast cancer in mammograms very accurately—without AI. Humans are very confident in their ability to predict, but when this is evaluated with rigorous science, their accuracy and consistency (intra-rater reliability) often do not match their confidence.[4] Figure 8.1 shows the results of a study in which

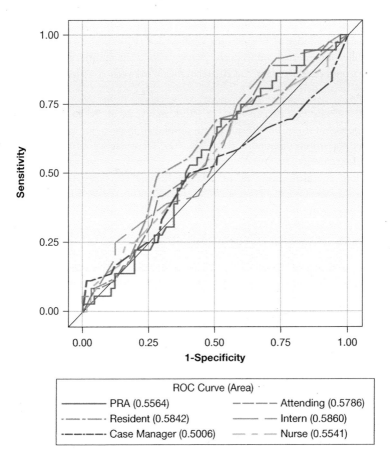

FIGURE 8.1. Inability of providers to predict unplanned readmissions. This study demonstrated that clinicians were unable to predict hospital readmissions. Gathering preliminary data like these can demonstrate the need for a predictive model. PRA is Probability of Repeat Admission, a standardized risk tool. (From Allaudeen N, Schnipper JL, Orav EJ, et al. Inability of providers to predict unplanned readmissions. *J Gen Intern Med.* 2011;26(7):771–776, with permission.)

people were asked to estimate the probability that a patient would be readmitted to the hospital. As you can see, they did not do much better than flipping a coin.

Change the AI culture from "eminence-based medicine" to "evidence-based medicine"

When proposing the development of an AI predictive model, having data on the ability and accuracy of prediction by skilled clinicians—without AI—is priceless. If at all possible, measure this first. Suppose you were developing a predictive model of postpartum hemorrhage (PPH). You could collect the following information from the providers for a few months and use it to report predictive accuracy and the relationship between confidence and the ability to predict.

1. Please rate this patient's risk of PPH on a scale of 0% to 100% (We know that it can be difficult to put a number on risk, but for this project please enter a number from 0 to 100, otherwise we cannot use this information.)
2. How confident are you in this prediction? (1—Very unconfident; 2—Unconfident 3—Neutral; 4—Confident; 5—Very confident)
3. What is your position? (1—attending, 2—resident, etc)
4. Type of delivery? (0—vaginal, 1—cesarean) Collect the outcome data:
5. Did this patient have PPH? (0—no, 1—yes)

This will enable you to create a receiver-operating-characteristics (ROC) curve and a calibration plot to show the difference between your predictive model and the clinicians' estimated probability.

The data from the questions above can also be used to assess the relationship between confidence and the ability to predict. Suppose that you collected these data and showed that the area under the receiver-operating-characteristic curve (AUC) was only 0.52 for clinicians. And suppose that you were able to create a predictive model that had an AUC of 0.81. This would be valuable information for implementation, a paper, and a grant application. The ROC graph with two lines for the AUCs of 0.52 and 0.81 would be the "money shot" for the project. Suppose that those with the highest confidence had the lowest ROCs. This is extremely valuable information in justifying the need for this model and this research.

The Dunning–Kruger effect is a cognitive bias stating that those with low ability at a task overestimate their own ability, and that those with high ability at a task underestimate their own ability.

> *"People hold overly favorable views of their abilities in many social and intellectual domains… this overestimation occurs, in part, because people who are unskilled in these domains suffer a dual burden: Not only do these people reach erroneous conclusions and make unfortunate choices, but their incompetence robs them of the metacognitive ability to realize it."*[5]

—JUSTIN KRUGER AND DAVID DUNNING.

From Kruger J, Dunning D. Unskilled and unaware of it: how difficulties in recognizing one's own incompetence lead to inflated self-assessments. *J Pers Soc Psychol.* 1999;77(6):1121-1134. Copyright © 1999, American Psychological Association, with permission.

> *"Our minds are susceptible to systematic errors in thinking caused by the design of the machinery of cognition not by corruption of thought or emotion."*

—DANIEL KAHNEMAN, 2002 NOBEL LAUREATE.[4]

To overcome the resistance to randomization, a successful technique is to start by randomizing in a small way but plan to expand when the clinicians are ready to adopt.

Identify only the top two patients at highest risk each day in the hospital. Then have the implementation team randomly select one of these patients and silently assess whether the known prevention measures were completed. A project that is new and complex may overwhelm the operations team, which is the "effector arm" of AI implementation. Therefore, a good approach is to start so small that it is impossible to resist. Run it silently and allow them to adjust and accept the AI tool. When they are comfortable, they will ask to expand it.

PRINCIPLE 83 • Improving outcomes does not have to be "5 years down the road."

Researchers discover a gene related to a disease or create a predictive model of a complication, or find a biomarker for a type of cancer; they publish a paper, advance their careers, and move on to another paper. When you ask about using their finding to improve health outcomes, the answer is often "That is 5 years down the road." When you come back in 5, 10, or 15 years you will hear the same answer, but these people have advanced in their careers, so you cannot blame people for doing what they are incentivized to do. The solution is to realign the incentives.

> ### *i* FOR MORE INFORMATION
>
> Overcoming resistance to artificial intelligence projects. Mark Kirby.[6]

CHAPTER SUMMARY

Within medicine, we are simultaneously in the age of AI implementation and in the age of AI resistance. Overcoming the resistance requires using emotional intelligence and having a game plan. The AI project must be led by a clinician who is motivated to use AI to improve outcomes and is willing to randomize and accept the results of that experiment. Success also requires hiring skilled informatic professionals to export data sets in a format that can be easily used to build and validate models and to code the model back into the electronic health record.

Many in health care have a can't-do attitude regarding randomization of AI tools in pragmatic trials. Resistance also comes in the form of "we already do this." But when one examines the facts, this is often false. Many people have a "we already proved that this approach works" regarding the application of AI in medicine. The job of a modern health care leader is to diplomatically help them overcome these attitudes and guide them to success. Often progress in implementing AI in medicine is not about the performance of the models—it is about health care tribalism and turf battles. Leaders must help them transcend these problems to work together as a collaborative team.

Health care is a competitive field and those who are late adopters of AI may find that it is difficult to catch up to those who invested early. Successful health care organizations will disrupt their old product or service with a superior one based on AI before someone else does it for them. Become Uber—don't become Ubered! But don't become Theronos and don't become Theronosed.

REFERENCES

1. Williamson P. Take the time and effort to correct misinformation. *Nature*. 2016;540(7632):171.
2. Ambasciano L. *Ghosts, post-truth despair, and Brandolini's Law. An Unnatural History of Religions: Academia, Post-truth and the Quest for Scientific Knowledge.* Bloomsbury Publishing; 2018:11.

3. Thatcher J, Shears A, Eckert J. *Rethinking the geoweb and big data: mixed methods and Brandolini's Law. Thinking Big Data in Geography: New Regimes, New Research.* University of Nebraska Press; 2018:232. ISBN 978-1-4962-0537-7. doi:10.2307/j.ctt21h4z6m.

4. Kahneman D. *Thinking, Fast and Slow. Farrar, Straus and Giroux.* New York; 2011.

5. Kruger J, Dunning D. Unskilled and unaware of it: how difficulties in recognizing one's own incompetence lead to inflated self-assessments. *J Pers Soc Psychol.* 1999;77(6):1121-1134.

6. Kirby M. Overcoming resistance to artificial intelligence projects. https://www.youtube.com/watch?v=P15CQ03eLcQ

CHAPTER 9

Execution—
Increasing the Odds of Future Success

A top priority for any high-performance health care system is to generate actionable insights from data—in a timely manner. AI tools are currently available to deliver on this, but there is much implementation work to be done.

> *"The question has changed from: 'IF, to HOW, AI will impact health outcomes?'"*
>
> —Lily Peng, Physician-scientist, Google Health.

PRINCIPLE 84 • Use Adaptive Platform Trials (APTs) to assess specific forms implementation.[1]

Adaptive platform prospective patient-level randomized controlled trials (RCTs) are often the ideal way to study many AI tools in health care (Figure 9.1). An APT is an RCT in which multiple interventions can be tested and multiple questions can be answered in parallel. These trials are ideal for AI implementation because they allow one to be adaptive and test multiple AI implementations, drop the loser arm for futility, keep the winner, and add new arms in a perpetual manner without long delays between studies. The arms change based on a prespecified decision algorithm in the master protocol. Likewise, the study can also adapt to change the randomization ratio based on findings from the study.

Adaptive platform trial designs should be used to evaluate a number of AI implementation options simultaneously and efficiently. The RCT forces researchers and care teams to clearly prespecify and define their interventions and outcomes and then gives the ability to modify the intervention until the outcome improves.

As you adapt, focus on improving a specific patient outcome based on an effect made by a change in clinician behavior.

Some are concerned that APTs are too complex, but this requires a change in one's mindset. Rather than assessing whether a specific strategy

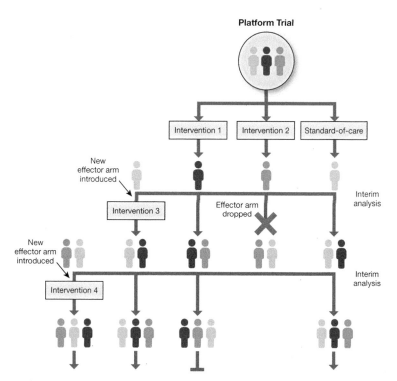

FIGURE 9.1. Adaptive Platform Trial (APT) study design. For AI tools to improve patient outcomes, there needs to be an effector arm. Since the first iteration of an effector arm may not be successful, the APT provides a nimble method of stopping an approach that is not working and staring a new approach. (Reprinted from Park JJH, Harari O, Dron L, Lester RT, Thorlund K, Mills EJ. An overview of platform trials with a checklist for clinical readers. *J Clin Epidemiol.* 2020;125:1-8, with permission from Elsevier.)

reduces the rate of a complication with a yes or no answer, the APT trial focuses on how to reduce the rate of a complication. In year 1, one might try A vs usual care, and if A is found to be better, the trial adapts to compare A vs B, and so on.

PRINCIPLE 85 • **After creating an AI tool, focus on creating and testing an <u>effector arm</u> in a pragmatic trial.**

Many AI researchers are incentivized to create and publish new models. **In fact, there is almost an arms race to build a model with a higher area**

under the receiver-operating-characteristic curve (AUC). Yet, most of those models are never used to improve patient outcomes because they lack an effector arm—an intervention or plan to intervene.

An effector arm is the implementation intervention that takes the information from the AI tool and makes a meaningful behavioral change which seeks to improve patient outcomes. For example, a hematologist prioritized the patients identified to be at highest risk for a blood clot and ensures that the patients receive the appropriate prophylaxis. The effector arm might be that a pressure injury prevention nurse rounds on those identified to be at highest risk to ensure that the pressure injury prevention steps are taken. The effector arm might be that patients who have a high risk of breast cancer from an AI mammogram tool are double-checked by a radiologist.

Many AI projects fail because of the difficulty of creating and sustaining an effector arm. One should not underestimate how difficult this can be to accomplish in a busy fragmented hospital. Health care leaders from multiple domains are required to work together to enact an effector arm. The algorithm must do more than provide a probability, score, or colored alert. The system must provide a simple evidence-based actionable prompt—that is acted upon.

Why are AI models rarely tested in RCTs? In the race to improve the AUC, researchers often create models that can never be used in practice because they use factors that are not available in real time. Many include factors that are based on reverse causation—one of the predictors is actually the result of the outcome. Smokers often quit smoking when they learn they have lung cancer and therefore ex-smoker is a "predictor" of lung cancer. People who develop gout stop exercising and therefore being sedentary "predicts" gout. Complications that result in a laboratory test ordered or drug prescribed can easily be "misinterpreted" by a black box proprietary algorithm with a large number of features.

For some AI applications, the implementation needs to be centralized to one person or team that is responsible and accountable.

The idea of educating every doctor and nurse about a new AI tool and how they should do their jobs differently is unlikely to be successful. The hope that they will all be convinced of the statistical properties of the model is a formula for failure. Alternatively, educate, convince, and prepare a small team that is supportive of the approach. Then together identify the obstacles for the effector arm and test if outcomes improve.

"Those who cannot remember the past are condemned to repeat it."

—GEORGE SANTAYANA.

The AI model is not a "magic bullet." Understanding how physicians make decisions in the clinical workflow and implementing AI tools seamlessly with an effector arm is the key to success.

Health care systems will need to change the incentives and reward implementation teams who move a project along in a way that changes clinicians' actions and demonstrates that the model is not only accurate but is improving health.

> *"Designing and implementing effector arms that induce meaningful behavior change will be the key to AI moving from the hype stage to one in which is it contributing to meaningful improvements in health and health care."*[2]

—Ezekiel Emanuel and Robert Wachter.

Clinical decision support alerts

PRINCIPLE 86 • **Interventions based solely on alerts in the electronic health record (EHR) are nearly always failures. Some of the best AI solutions are the ones that work in the background, appear to be routine, pedestrian, and taken for granted.**

When one looks for examples of successful alerts in everyday life that have improved health of a large population in a cost-effective and sustainable manner, one of the best examples is the seat belt warning alert. The unused seat belt has no value. The ignored alert has no value. But the alert that changes behavior has value—a safer passenger (Table 9.1).

Obviously, simply showing a score in the EHR will not improve patient outcomes, if it does not change clinician behavior. If everyone continues to do their job the same way, even the most accurate and precise predictive model will have no impact.

First deliver, then promise what you can do with AI.

Building highly customized effector arm solutions in health care will take time. The AI tool can provide valuable decision support about risk, but clinicians must decide how to treat the high-risk patients. AI tools are generally very weak at identifying what the high-risk patient needs. Some AI projects fail because they attempt to have the computer do both parts of this work.

The effector arm is the plan that clinicians will enact to use the risk stratification information. This work takes time and unrealistic promises

TABLE 9.1	Clinical Decision Support vs Seat Belt Alerts	
	Seat Belt	**Most Clinical Decision Support**
Does it alert the user in a smart way?	Y	N
If ignored, is there an effective escalation?	Y	N
Does the user change their behavior based on the alert?	Y	N
Does this change in behavior result in improved health outcomes for a large population?	Y	N
Is there a good return on investment for this alert?	Y	N
Is the alert and change in behavior scalable and sustainable?	Y	N

about the timelines hurt credibility, so rather than promising broad ambitious AI projects that will be completed quickly, start small. Carefully pick the right problem to solve and build on that success. Pick a feasible AI project that creates value for the users, like improving a core operation in an important way. Have an experienced team define the right project. Then deliver a quick win and use that to gain momentum. Under promise and over deliver.

Focus on successfully improving one health outcome with AI in a narrow area and then expand on this success.

Much of the failure in the past has come from overly ambitious broad AI projects in health care. Instead consider the Steve Jobs approach. Each year Jobs would meet with his team and list 10 potential projects that they could work on, and then force them boil it down to 3 that they could achieve with excellence. This focus was a key to his success.

Think GPS—not self-driving car. Provide value to physicians—do not try to replace them. Start with AI technology that is ripe and marry that to a problem that unleashes clinical benefit. Understand the pain points in the current clinical workflow and health care system. Ideally, you will have a physician lead the project who can gain internal allies and with success in specific niches; it will expand to health care–wide core practices.

PRINCIPLE 87 • Compute the power and sample size to ensure that you will have a sufficient number of patients to assess improvement.

Basic statistical planning is necessary for a study of impact including through consideration of the number of patients you will need to build and validate a model and how many are necessary to assess the model's impact. Rather than describing these statistical principles in this book, please see Chapter 9 of "Publishing Your Medical Research" to learn more about this.[3] Then gather sufficient preliminary data to work with the biostatistician on your team. Provide information on the amount of patient data and the percent of patients potentially impacted.

For an impact study, you will need to know the current rate of the event, the number of patients per year that meets the inclusion criteria, and some estimate of what a clinically meaningful improvement in the rate of the outcome would be. Researching the sample sizes of publications that have attempted to answer the research question is also valuable. Models for hospital-wide conditions should ideally be assessed across the entire hospital. This enables having the statistical power to detect an impact in less than a year in most cases. Models generally cannot be efficiently assessed in just one unit of the hospital because of the small sample size.

PRINCIPLE 88 • Consider creating two models to allow clinicians to balance the probabilities of benefit and harm for the intervention.

For example, the probability of a venous thromboembolism and the probability of bleeding could be displayed for a patient, and this could be stratified with prophylaxis vs without prophylaxis. This information would provide clinical decision support (CDS) for the physicians allowing them to weigh the pros and cons of administering venous thromboembolism prophylaxis for a given patient. Another example of the two-model approach is to provide the probability of good outcomes if the patient were given saline vs a balanced crystalloid. The models should be based on RCT, not observational, data, for example from studies like CLOT or SMART[4,5] (Figure 9.2).

	Without VTE prophylaxis	**With VTE prophylaxis**
Probability of a blood clot	23%	3%
Probability of bleeding	<1%	2%

FIGURE 9.2. Counterfactual probabilities, clotting, and bleeding, with and without venous thromboembolism (VTE) prophylaxis. This is a hypothetical example used to illustrate how four predictive models could be used to provide information to clinicians to help them make optimal decisions.

PRINCIPLE 89 • **To be successful at the implementation of AI in medicine, learn from previous failures and study the "Valley of Death" where AI models died (Table 9.2).**

TABLE 9.2	**Common Themes of AI Failures**

Overpromising.

Not explaining how the models work.

Failing to understand the clinical workflow and the needs of the users.

Having nonphysicians lead the project.

Ignoring the importance of obtaining buy-in from nursing.

Expecting that a simple alert would change behavior.

Creating "friction-full" clinical decision support.

PRINCIPLE 90 • **Pragmatic clinical trials provide the opportunity to assess clinical decision support.**

We conducted a pragmatic RCT to assess the impact of an alert based on real-time prediction for acute kidney injury among hospitalized pediatric patients. For the intensive care patients, among those at risk, more serum creatinine tests were ordered for the intervention group than for controls (69% vs 60%, $P = .002$).[6] This study demonstrated that it was possible to randomize all of the patients in a pediatric hospital and assess an AI tool. It also demonstrated that an alert based on a predictive model could be used to improve the rate of ordering a clinically important test. Larger studies are required to determine the impact of increased screening on clinical outcomes such as acute kidney injury incidence and severity.

PRINCIPLE 91 • Successful implementation of an AI tool is often accomplished by having a dedicated person or small team review the high-risk patients on a worklist rather than trying to train and change thousands of busy clinicians.

Showing the probability for one patient to one clinician at a time may not be the best approach. A report that sorts all patients in the hospital by their risk may be more useful. For many projects, simply displaying the probability in the EHR or using an alert/BPA (best practice alert) is ineffective. For many projects, a more effective approach is to have an implementation/installation plan that will include a project bundle and a multicomponent intervention. For patients at the highest risk, the known prevention steps will be triple checked to ensure that they are performed in a timely way. Simplify the work process and ensure that there is reliable execution.

BPAs or CDS alerts are ignored much of the time.[7,8] Alert fatigue, caused by the computer crying wolf, causes clinical frustration. An alert is a simplistic solution that by itself is often insufficient. AI implementation requires the addition of a reward to consistently change behavior. Alerts should have a thank you factor. What is the reward for the person who responds to the alert?

> *"Clinical trials of seemingly benign interventions, such as alerts, require rigorous evaluation and should not be implemented without robust evidence of safety and efficacy."*
>
> —Wilson et al[9]

 FOR MORE INFORMATION

RE-AIM and PRISM—"an integrated framework developed to improve the adoption and sustainable implementation of evidence-based interventions in a wide range of health, public health, educational, community, and other settings."[10]
PS: Power and Sample Size Calculation (free software). William D. Dupont and Walton D. Plummer, Jr https://biostat.app.vumc.org/wiki/Main/PowerSampleSize.

CHAPTER SUMMARY

This chapter brings together the best of many clinical and analytic fields to create a recipe for success. This requires understanding the strengths and weaknesses of each domain. We need the rigor of science without the inefficiencies of science. We need the can-do attitude and resources of industry without the weak evaluations of industry. We are in the age of AI implementation and our health care system must provide incentives to move AI breakthroughs to follow-throughs.

Understand and empathize with the clinicians who are very smart and experienced. They have been identifying high-risk patients and diagnosing diseases for years and they will not easily accept that an AI tool will replace their judgment. So, build a solution that is frictionless and makes their work easier with augmented intelligence amplification. The computerized physician order entry system is often the ideal point in the workflow to test AI. Education alone about AI models does not change health outcomes. Clinician and/or patient behaviors must also change.

Focus on a specific problem that AI can add value to and test with randomization. Do not let the marketing people overpromise what AI can do in health care. Have the technical people accurately describe what is feasible and have the scientists describe what the studies proved. Translate AI discovery into health by applying knowledge to extend life and improve the quality of life.

Balance scientific and statistical rigor with pragmatism. The attitude that "It is never good enough" causes delays and gets theoretical perfectionists marginalized. Successful applied AI researchers know when to pick their battles and avoid being overly critical when it does not matter. For many AI applications in health care, the model performance is not the issue. The implementation and randomized pragmatic controlled trial are what matter.

REFERENCES

1. Adaptive Platform Trials Coalition. Adaptive platform trials: definition, design, conduct and reporting considerations. *Nat Rev Drug Discov.* 2019;18(10):797-807. Erratum in: *Nat Rev Drug Discov.* 2019 10.
2. Emanuel EJ, Wachter RM. Artificial Intelligence in health care: will the value match the hype? *JAMA.* 2019;321(23):2281-2282.
3. Byrne D. *Publishing Your Medical Research.* Wolters Kluwer; 2017. https://www.slideshare.net/DanielByrne12/publishing-your-medical-research-125452257

4. Walker SC, Creech CB, Domenico HJ, French B, Byrne DW, Wheeler AP. A real-time risk-prediction model for pediatric venous thromboembolic events. *Pediatrics*. 2021;147(6):e2020042325.
5. Semler MW, Self WH, Wanderer JP, et al. Balanced crystalloids versus saline in critically ill adults. *N Engl J Med*. 2018;378(9):829-839.
6. Van Driest SL, Wang L, McLemore MF, et al. Acute kidney injury risk-based screening in pediatric inpatients: a pragmatic randomized trial. *Pediatr Res*. 2020;87(1):118-124.
7. Lehman CD, Wellman RD, Buist DSM, et al. Diagnostic accuracy of digital screening mammography with and without computer-aided detection. *JAMA Intern Med*. 2015;175:1828-1837.
8. Phansalkar S, van der Sijs H, Tucker AD, et al. Drug-drug interactions that should be non-interruptive in order to reduce alert fatigue in electronic health records. *J Am Med Inf Assoc*. 2013;20:489-493.
9. Wilson FP, Martin M, Yamamoto Y, et al. Electronic health record alerts for acute kidney injury: multicenter, randomized clinical trial. *BMJ*. 2021; 372:m4786.
10. RE-AIM working group. RE-AIM and PRISM. https://re-aim.org/

CHAPTER 10

Integration— Building a Learning Health Care System With Pragmatic AI Trials

PRINCIPLE 92 • "Big data" alone are inadequate to address the effectiveness of medical interventions like AI tools.

A learning health care system implements rigorous science to improve patient outcomes based on lessons learned during routine clinical care. The learning health care system provides a framework in which to test an aspect of medicine, or an aspect of a core operation that has yet to be truly shown, in an evidenced-based manner, to be the most effective option. Clinical equipoise is defined as a genuine uncertainty over whether an intervention or treatment will be beneficial. The learning health care system has successfully tested these aspects of medical care.

Most Artificial Intelligence (AI) projects are implementing a new predictive model with an effector arm to change clinical behavior. Uncertainty about whether it will be more beneficial than harmful certainly exists, so the learning health care system framework can support this work as well. Rather than perpetuating uncertainty with untested AI tools, we must conduct such pragmatic randomized controlled trials (RCTs) to be evidence based.

When addressing the effectiveness of AI interventions into clinical care, big data are not a substitute for pragmatic randomized trials in a learning health care system. Although there is much talk about big data as an alternative, most people are unaware of the serious limitations of the observational studies which contribute to big data. Table 10.1 illustrates a few examples in which we have found conflicting conclusions between published observational studies and our randomized pragmatic trials. Others have shown how randomized trials can produce very different conclusions than similar observational studies.[8]

TABLE 10.1	Examples Illustrating the Differences Between Random and Nonrandom Studies	
Research Question	**Nonrandomized Studies**	**Randomized Studies**
1. Chlorhexidine. Does daily bathing with chlorhexidine reduce hospital-acquired infections?	Yes[1]	No[2]
2. Postdischarge phone calls. Does a postdischarge phone call reduce hospital readmissions and improve patient satisfaction?	Yes[3]	No[4]
3. SMART/SALT-ED Are balanced crystalloid IV fluids, such as lactated Ringer's solution, safer than saline?	No[5]	Yes[6,7]

PRINCIPLE 93 • Pragmatic trials are efficient ways to assess the real-world impact of AI tools in medicine.

A pragmatic RCT is a study that assesses the impact of a treatment or intervention on a patient outcome in a real-world health care system during routine care. This differs from a clinical trial in which volunteers are recruited and the study is performed in a controlled environment, such as a clinical research center. A pragmatic trial is less expensive than other trials in that it uses routinely collected data during clinical care. In fact, the ideal study design for AI is often one that is frictionless. Peter Pronovost, the patient safety champion, describes a collaborative model to move discoveries into practice. He teaches how to learn from health care integration success stories and describes several pragmatic trials in practice.[9] Those working to implement AI in a clinical workflow can learn from his success stories. For those who are not quite ready to test their AI tool in a pragmatic trial, Sachs et al provide "a framework for emulating a prediction-driven trial to evaluate the clinical utility of a prediction-based decision rule in observational data."[10] This preliminary work may provide the evidence to gain support to conduct an actual RCT.

PRINCIPLE 94 • Plan for an iterative approach. The first implementation with the AI tool is unlikely to improve patient outcomes; perhaps the second or third approach will.

Everyone knows the story of Thomas Edison who made 1000 unsuccessful attempts at inventing the light bulb. When a reporter asked, "How did it feel to fail 1000 times?" Edison replied, "I didn't fail 1000 times. The light bulb was an invention with 1000 steps." Failure plays such an important role in innovation that there is now a "Museum of Failure" that celebrates the learning experience of failure.[11]

Once an AI model is developed, the effector arm needs to be tested with the Edison approach—keep trying various iterations until we get it right. Does an alert work? Is a dedicated central rounding team needed? Does there need to be an escalation for ignored alerts? Failure is acceptable when we learn from it. Therefore, the adaptive platform trial design works well.

Develop an efficient process to support AI projects for a learning healthcare system

AI projects in health care should be supported by hospital leaders if the team agrees to (1) randomize the new AI tool and compare to usual care, (2) use a primary end point of improving an important patient outcome, and (3) submit the results for publication. The projects should earn support if they build on previous work to continue on the march of progress. Our health care system needs leaders who are not afraid to support multiple attempts for this progress. Is there a previous project that the team could improve upon? Are there teams already working on this that could be collaborators?

> *"Fortune favors the brave."*
> —Latin proverb.

PRINCIPLE 95 • Learn why intention-to-treat (ITT) analysis is essential for discovering the correct conclusion.

ITT analysis is a method of analyzing results from an RCT in which all patients are included in the arm to which they were randomized, regardless of whether or not they received the treatment. Although this may seem counterintuitive to some, this is the proper way to draw conclusions about the larger research question. For example, an AI model predicts a risk score for condition X. Patients in the hospital are randomly assigned to two groups. Both groups include patients with varying stages of risk. Those in group 1 (high and low risk) receive all of the usual care procedures offered but the physician is not aware of the risk score. In group 2, all of the patients (high and low risk) receive the usual care procedures offered but the physician is made aware of those that have the highest risk scores and uses this information to prioritize rounding and an effector arm ensures they receive preventive care (usual care plus a predictive model of risk).

Once the study is completed, the ITT analysis will compare all of the patients from both groups, the low-risk and high-risk patients in groups 1 and 2. The analysis will reveal if this AI tool's risk stratification led to improved patient outcomes, compared with usual care alone. The non-ITT approach answers a trivial question "Are the patients who were intervened on different from the control group?"

Note that the ITT approach was used in all the randomized studies in Table 10.1. One of those studies assessed whether a postdischarge phone call program reduced hospital readmissions. Patients were randomized into two groups: usual care vs usual care plus postdischarge phone call. A nurse attempted to call all of the patients in the intervention arm after they were discharged from the hospital but was only able to reach 59% of them. Since only these patients received the intervention, many flawed studies would base the analysis on this subset vs the control group. This gives the wrong answer to the study question "Does a postdischarge phone call program reduce readmissions?" The answer to that question can only be found by using the ITT approach of comparing all of the patients randomized to the control arm to all of the patients randomized to the intervention arm. The patients who answered the phone were different from those who did not answer the phone in every way measured. Some patients did not answer the phone because they had already been readmitted to the hospital, demonstrating the fundamental flaw in that analysis.

PRINCIPLE 96 • Assess that you have separation between the intervention group and the control group. Assess whether there is learning in the control group.

With pragmatic clinical trial study designs, some are worried that the use of a model will influence the care of patients in the control group. Contamination, or cross-over, can occur if clinicians learn to identify high-risk patients based on what they learn from the model, and this influences them to also identify and treat high-risk patients in the control arm. This would bias the results toward the null, meaning that an effective intervention would appear to be less effective than it truly is. A larger sample size will not fix this problem but will enable you to detect smaller differences. In our experience, hospitals are so busy with so many moving parts that this contamination rarely happens, but this should be evaluated.

How do you assure that you are getting separation between the control and intervention groups? Is it possible that the people applying the interventional "extra care" will consciously or unconsciously up their vigilance/diligence for all patients who fit their intuitive mold, even if they do not see the risk scores for all patients? When planning a pragmatic trial, it is wise to plan to mitigate this but also measure for these types of problems, but this is not a good reason to downgrade from a strong patient-level randomized pragmatic trial to a weaker study design.

TABLE 10.2 A Comparison of the Current Health Care System vs a New Health Care System That Uses AI in an Optimal Way	
The Current Health Care Without AI	**New Learning Health Care System With AI**
One-size-fits-all	Personalized medicine
Manual scoring systems of risk	Automated risk stratification
Reactive	Proactive (predicting and preventing)
Managed with lagging indicators	Managed with leading indicators
Conditions caught downstream	Conditions caught upstream
Episodic	Population based
Wasteful/saddled with inefficiencies	More efficient
Costly	Less expensive
Eminence based	Evidence based
Gestalt/best guess	Precise prediction
Patients/families excluded	Patients/families are engaged
Burns out clinicians	Reduces the work of clinicians

PRINCIPLE 97 • Incentives in health care should be realigned to move to a new health care system that uses and tests AI in an optimal way (Table 10.2).

It is healthy to be idealistic, but the reality is that people do what they are incentivized to do. Academic promotions should reward multidisciplinary teamwork and publications that demonstrate that patient outcomes were improved—or at least assessed. Industry career promotions should reward those who complete rigorous evaluations. Financial incentives for hospitals and physicians should always prioritize patient outcomes but especially for AI implementation projects. AI implementation research requires being an optimist but also a pragmatist.

Funding agencies such as NIH, CMS, and PCORI and policy-makers should increase the grant applications announcements that encourage randomization of AI tools. In the past, these agencies have sometimes discouraged the use of randomization, which has wasted enormous amounts of taxpayer money. The Request For Application should insist on projects that are true advances of AI implementation.

Insurance companies, the FDA, Joint Commission, Occupational Safety and Health Administration, the U.S. News & World Report, ANCC Magnet Recognition Program, and CMS's Star Ratings, can all play a role in creating incentives to use and evaluate AI tools with rigor to benefit patients. These organizations can also create healthy AI competitions that would move the field forward. This could be similar to the protein folding CASP competition that the DeepMind AlphaFold team recently won. See Chapter 15 for more details about AlphaFold.

 FOR MORE INFORMATION

Museum of Failure. Samuel West.[11] https://museumoffailure.com/

CHAPTER SUMMARY

Do not accept the idea that health care is the way it is and there is nothing you can do about it. By changing incentives to encourage rigorous evaluations of AI implementation, the technology can start to have an impact. The learning health care system framework can support pragmatic RCTs during routine care. An adaptive platform trial design allows for a team to assess multiple types of implementation simultaneously.

REFERENCES

1. Duszyńska W, Adamik B, Lentka-Bera K, et al. Effect of universal chlorhexidine decolonisation on the infection rate in intensive care patients. *Anaesthesiol Intensive Ther*. 2017;49(1):28-33.

2. Noto MJ, Domenico HJ, Byrne DW, et al. Chlorhexidine bathing and health care-associated infections: a randomized clinical trial. *JAMA*. 2015;313(4):369-378.

3. Chestnut VM, Vadyak K, McCambridge MM, Weiss MJ. The impact of telephonic follow-up within 2 business days postdischarge on 30-day readmissions for patients with heart failure. *J Dr Nurs Pract*. Published online January 19, 2021:JDNP-D-19-00079. doi: 10.1891/JDNP-D-19-00079.

4. Yiadom MYAB, Domenico HJ, Byrne DW, et al. Impact of a follow-up telephone call program on 30-day readmissions (FUTR-30): a pragmatic randomized controlled real-world effectiveness trial. *Med Care*. 2020;58(9):785-792.

5. Rochwerg B, Alhazzani W, Gibson A, et al. Fluid type and the use of renal replacement therapy in sepsis: a systematic review and network meta-analysis. *Intensive Care Med*. 2015;41(9):1561-1571.

6. Semler MW, Self WH, Wanderer JP, et al. Balanced crystalloids versus saline in critically ill adults. *N Engl J Med*. 2018;378(9):829-839.

7. Self WH, Semler MW, Wanderer JP, et al. Balanced crystalloids versus saline in noncritically ill adults. *N Engl J Med*. 2018;378(9):819-828.

8. Young SS, Karr A. Deming, data and observational studies. A process out of control and needing fixing. *Significance*. 2011;9:122-126.

9. Pronovost PJ, Berenholtz SM, Needham DM. Translating evidence into practice: a model for large scale knowledge translation. *BMJ*. 2008;337:a1714.

10. Sachs MC, Sjölander A, Gabriel EE. Aim for clinical utility, not just predictive accuracy. *Epidemiology*. 2020;31(3):359-364.

11. West S. Museum of failure. Samuel West. https://museumoffailure.com/

11

Streamlining— Reducing Waste and Lowering Costs in Health Care

PRINCIPLE 98 • Prevention of disease and complications from illness will lower costs.

The most widely accepted approach to lowering health care costs is to reduce waste associated with preventable problems.[1] Advances in Artificial Intelligence (AI) allow us, for the first time, to predict many complications and diseases with a high level of accuracy and precision. This improvement in predictive efficiency will become central to a health care organization's survival.

Approximately 30% of the U.S. health care system is waste, which is more than $750 billion per year in the United States. These are expenses that add no value. At forward-thinking health care organizations, the money wasted in these areas will be identified with modern science and moved into resources that add value, such as prevention and wellness, new AI approaches and resources, and cost savings for patients. This level of waste is obviously unsustainable and therefore institutions that use AI to reduce this waste will have a huge competitive advantage.

Approximately 90% of the U.S. health care system is still fee-for-service, where physicians and hospitals are paid more to do more. As the system changes to more value-based reimbursement, pressure will be applied to use AI tools. As payers move to these value-based or capitation payment models, hospitals will absorb the cost of hospital stays delayed by complications and they will be penalized for preventable health problems.

Hospitals are already penalized for readmission rates that are excessive, but most have floundered at implementing predictive models which can be used to prevent avoidable readmissions. Payers have the data, and the payments will be based on results not on false claims from flawed evaluations, such as those in Table 2.3. Without the accurate risk prediction from AI, hospitals will not be able to focus scarce prevention resources. Without testing

165

the implementation with a randomized controlled trial, hospitals will not learn what form of implementation improves outcomes for those at high risk.

PRINCIPLE 99 • Predictive analytics are successfully being used to detect and reduce medical fraud and abuse.

Models are being used to sort health claims by the probability that they are fraudulent. Then humans review the subset of claims with the highest probability rather than all of them. This saves money by reducing the number of people needed to review claims and is an area in which AI is very precise, accurate, and adds value. The models can also be used to detect patient fraud, upcoding, criminal networks, and kickbacks.

PRINCIPLE 100 • AI tools can be used to reduce waste by focusing laboratory screening where it is needed most.

Some laboratory test results are predictable, making ordering them costly and sometimes unnecessary. Jonathan Chen, a physician-scientist at Stanford, has demonstrated that showing physicians the probability that a laboratory test would most likely be normal reduces unnecessary testing.[2]

On the other hand, AI can be used for pre-emptive testing by predicting that a laboratory test value would be abnormal. For example, some tests are likely to be abnormal and actionable, for example, a complete blood count (CBC), basic metabolic panel (BMP), troponin level, lipid panel, or a serum albumin test. Predictive models can prompt physicians to order a test that is both likely to be abnormal and actionable.

Alerts can prompt clinicians to order additional tests or enter additional information that is required to compute the model with better precision. For example, while one would assume that serum albumin which is a very strong predictor of pressure injuries would be ordered on admission, it is missing for 80% of patients. An AI algorithm could predict if albumin was abnormal. Ordering it would then improve the precision of the pressure injury model. Similar models could be developed for more general tests such as the CBC or BMP (Figure 11.1).

PRINCIPLE 101 • Focus on automating administrative tasks to reduce the workload of hospital administrators as well as nurses and physicians.

Many administrative tasks are routine and involve prediction, which are ripe for automation with an AI tool. Although early implementation of AI tools

This patient has a 93% probability of undiagnosed
Type 2 diabetes.

Click here to order a hemoglobin A1c test. [ ]

This probability is based on the following factors:

BMI	35.2
Age	58.2
Hypertension	Yes
Total Cholesterol	245
HDL	26
Smoking status	Current smoker

THIS ALERT DOES NOT FIRE FOR ALL PATIENTS.
This patient is part of a randomized trial.
For more information click here. [link].

FIGURE 11.1. Vaporware of pre-emptive testing. Predictive models can
identify patients who have undiagnosed conditions, such as Type 2 diabetes.
Their physician can be alerted and asked if they would like to order a hemoglobin A1c test. Although these models have been available for decades, the
challenge is how to incorporate them into routine care. Vaporware refers to a
mockup of what software could look like in the future.

should focus on improving patient outcomes, the funding for these projects needs to come from somewhere. Therefore, AI tools that save money
are also needed. Excessive medical administrative costs and complexity
are major problems that can be improved with AI. For every doctor in the
United States, there are nine administrative people. AI can help streamline
the administrative system in many ways (Table 11.1).

Randomization enables us to assess whether an AI tool or any health care
intervention adds value. If it does, keep it. If not, get rid of it. Daily bathing
with chlorhexidine, for example, is one such intervention (Table 10.1).[3] We
randomized 9340 ICU patients in a pragmatic trial to daily bathing with
chlorhexidine vs usual care and concluded that daily bathing with chlorhexidine did not reduce the incidence of health care–associated infections. The
challenge is that even after this study was completed and published in JAMA
there is tremendous resistance within the health care system to change. Many
hospitals continue with the unnecessary layer of work and expense, even
though proven to have no clinical value.

To avoid burning out clinicians, remove a layer of work before adding
another. No layer of AI work should be added without solid evidence of value

TABLE 11.1	Examples of How AI Can Reduce Waste

Predicting and preventing complications can attenuate the rate at which hospitals must absorb the cost of excessive lengths of stay due to complications.

Estimating the hospital discharge date.

Assessing the probability that a patient's discharge would be delayed or complex.

Reducing unnecessary readmissions.

Focusing limited resources on patients who need it most.

Identifying the right medication for each patient with precision medicine.

Scheduling patient visits in a smarter way by using empirical data, rather than triple booking patients and having them wait.

from a randomized controlled trial because AI tools should reduce the work of those in health care. Nurses and physicians have come to appreciate the value of randomized pragmatic trials for this reason.

AI can help hospitals in reducing the percent of health care claims that are denied. Insurance companies and Medicare often refuse to pay 10% to 15% of a hospital's claims. These nonpayments for services result in a major loss of income. A logistic regression model can compute probability of denial based on factors such as dollar amount of the claim (larger claims = more denials), days to submission, etc. Then claims can be sorted by probability of denial and attention can be applied to improve those large claims most likely to be denied.

PRINCIPLE 102 • Use AI tools to reduce patient wait times and improve satisfaction. Time to schedule new patient visits can be reduced with better analytics.

The probability that a given patient will show up for an appointment can be computed, reducing the need to triple book patients to account for "no shows." The sum of the probabilities can be used to estimate the number of patients to schedule and on average this should minimize patient wait times and maximize utilization. For example, if patient A has a 1.0 probability of showing up for their appointment, there is no over booking. If patients B and C each have a 0.5 probability of showing up, they are both scheduled for the same time. A "no show" model should avoid using predictors such as geographic indicators, health status, age, gender, race, or religion, which could cause ethical problems. Instead use predictors such as previous number of no shows and a pragmatic trial to randomize patients to usual care vs an AI system that schedules patients. The primary outcome would be wait times, secondary outcomes would be patient and staff satisfaction and the unit of analysis and randomization would probably be day rather than patient. Sensitivity analysis can also be performed to ensure that the new system is fair to all groups of patients.

> **ℹ FOR MORE INFORMATION**
>
> Application of Artificial Intelligence-Based Technologies in the Healthcare Industry: Opportunities and Challenges (Lee et al).[4]

> **CHAPTER SUMMARY**
>
> Health care has many potential areas in which AI utilization could identify waste, improve screening, testing, scheduling, and utilization. Moving these AI tools from a research project into a sustainable clinical workflow is the next step and will become essential for financial survival.

REFERENCES

1. Berwick DM, Hackbarth AD. Eliminating waste in U.S. health care. *JAMA.* 2012;307(14):1513-1516.
2. Xu S, Hom J, Balasubramanian S, et al. Prevalence and predictability of low-yield inpatient laboratory diagnostic tests. *JAMA Netw Open.* 2019;2(9):e1910967. Erratum in: *JAMA Netw Open.* 2019;2(10):e1914190.
3. Noto MJ, Domenico HJ, Byrne DW, et al. Chlorhexidine bathing and health care-associated infections: a randomized clinical trial. *JAMA.* 2015;313(4):369-378.
4. Lee D, Yoon SN. Application of artificial intelligence-based technologies in the healthcare industry: opportunities and challenges. *Int J Environ Res Publ Health.* 2021;18(1):271.

PART IV

The Specific Applications

Complications—Predicting and Preventing Hospital Complications

PRINCIPLE 103 • **Use AI tools to prevent complications before they happen.**

The myth that most hospital complications happen randomly and cannot be predicted has been disproven.[1] The myth that most complications cannot be prevented has been disproven.[2] Prevention, however, is generally most effective if focused on the high risk[3] which requires real-time automated risk stratification. Even with this, the first implementation approach that is attempted is unlikely to succeed—but the second or third might. The machinery of randomization shows us when the needle has moved.

Risk stratification, the process of separating patients by level of care needed, is an important application of Artificial Intelligence (AI) in medicine and learning to evaluate how well an AI tool provides risk stratification is an important skill. When evaluating a tool's ability to stratify risk, keep in mind that there are evaluation criteria for tools that are designed to stratify risk and prognosis and different evaluation criteria for tools that stratify for risk and diagnosis. In fact, the first step in building any predictive model is to carefully think about and discuss with your team what is the purpose of the model. Models created for real-time risk stratification will be completely different from models that are adjusting for confounding factors for a paper.

Obviously, simply creating an AI tool to predict hospital complications will not improve outcomes. Embedding the model into the electronic health record (EHR) and displaying the probability to physicians and nurses has little effect. Even if the AI tool is very accurate, if everyone continues to do their job in the same way, outcomes cannot improve (Figure 12.1).

For AI to succeed in medicine, some job roles must change. Prevention resources across the hospital must be allocated differently, using the information from the model to focus prevention where it is most needed. This change could be as simple as assigning one case manager to focus on

Complication	Risk on admission	Current risk
Pressure injury	15%	93%
Readmission	14%	15%
Acute kidney injury	7%	8%
Blood clot (venous thromboembolism)	2%	7%
Hospital acquired infection	2%	4%
Adverse drug event	1%	2%
Sepsis	1%	2%
Delirium	1%	1%
Fall in the hospital	1%	1%
ICU readmission	1%	1%
Pneumonia	1%	1%
Post-traumatic stress disorder	1%	1%
Unexpected death	1%	1%
Clostridioides difficile infection	0%	1%
Methicillin-resistant *Staphylococcus aureus* (MRSA) infection	0%	1%
Significant complication after surgery	2%	0%
Ventilator-associated pneumonia (VAP)	1%	0%
Catheter-associated urinary tract infection (CAUTI)	0%	0%
Central line bloodstream infection (CLABSI)	0%	0%
Surgical site infection	0%	0%
Need for hospice	0%	0%
Non-ICU cardiac arrest	0%	0%

FIGURE 12.1. Vaporware of a patient's risk of various complications sorted by probabilities. AI predictive models will be used to display risk of various hospital complications and rank them by importance to help focus limited hospital resources.

preventing readmissions in the patients in the intervention arm which showed the highest risk for return to hospital. This requires hospital leadership's support for a new approach and support for an evaluation with randomization. Sometimes there is resistance because leaders think this will require hiring new people but often it simply means that the same people work in a new way. In many cases, the AI tool removes the time-consuming work of manually identifying the high-risk patients and can reduce the workload by providing a more precise way to focus existing resources (Table 12.1).

PRINCIPLE 104 • Understand the difference between signal and noise.

A major problem in reducing hospital complications is a lack of understanding between signal and noise when evaluating rates over time. For example, see Figure 12.2. The signal is the truth, which can be seen with the long-trend

TABLE 12.1	AI Predictive Models That Could be Used to Reduce Hospital Complications

Acute kidney injury

Adverse drug events

Blood clots (venous thromboembolisms)

Delirium

Falls in the hospital and falls that required care and treatment

Hospital readmissions

Hypoxemia (low blood oxygen levels) 5 minutes before it happens in the OR[4]

ICU readmissions

Infections—Hospital Acquired

    Catheter-associated urinary tract infections

    Central line bloodstream infection

    Clostridioides difficile infection

    Methicillin-resistant *Staphylococcus aureus* infection

    Sepsis

    Surgical site infection

Mortality (at 28 days, 6 months, 1 year)

Need for hospice

Non-ICU cardiac arrests

Pneumonia

Post-traumatic stress disorder

Pressure injuries (pressure ulcers)

Significant complications after surgery

Unexpected death

Ventilator-associated pneumonia

line of the long run. The noise is based on short-term fluctuations. If one looks at a small window of time, the conclusion could be that patient falls are decreasing and interventions are working. If, however, one looks at the signal, the long-term pattern, the opposite conclusion is drawn. Falls are getting worse, and the prevention bundle is not working. Rigorous science and statistical analyses are the solution.

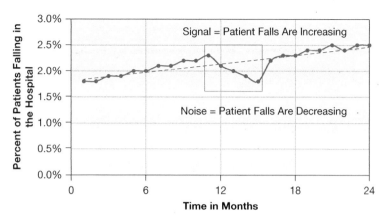

FIGURE 12.2. Whack-a-mole. The whack-a-mole approach focuses on the noise and results in clinician burnout and poor outcomes. The signal is the smoothed line. Hospital employees' incentives are often aligned with the whack-a-mole approach, but the incentives need to be changed to be aligned with long-term, sustainable improvement.

PRINCIPLE 105 • **Use predictive models to identify unexpected deaths and proactively focus prevention resources to reduce the observed to expected mortality.**

Obviously, some patients are admitted to the hospital in very poor health and are expected to die in the hospital. At the other extreme, there are patients who enter the hospital for a minor condition or procedure and die unexpectedly. AI tools can be used to identify these unexpected deaths based on data routinely collected on admission to the hospital—or at least in the first 24 hours. These probabilities of unexpected death can be updated every day based on new information for that patient, for example, laboratory data on day 2. The same model can be updated every day. There is no need to create a separate model with different predictors and coefficients for days 2, 3, and so on.

Every patient has an expected mortality (between 0 and 1) that is computed after discharge for the purposes of creating observed to expected mortality ratios. An average hospital will have an O:E of 1.0. Hospitals that are better than average and have fewer observed deaths than expected will have an O:E less than 1.0. Hospitals that are worse than average and have more deaths than expected have an O:E of more than 1.0.

We identified a group of patients with an expected mortality of less than 10%, who died during their hospital stay and defined these as "unexpected deaths." Then we built a predictive model of unexpected deaths from factors such as serum albumin, age, red cell distribution width, potassium, emergency department admission, blood urea nitrogen, mean corpuscular volume, hemoglobin, glucose, and male gender.

We sought to answer the question: "Which complete blood count laboratory values had a change from admission to the unexpected death (or discharge) that would be most predictive of the unexpected death?" The surprising answer was the red cell distribution width. The increase in the red cell distribution width was a strong predictor of an unexpected death.

How could this information be used to prevent the unexpected deaths? During rounds, the physicians could start with the patient with the highest probability. The patients with the highest probability of unexpected death could also serve as an important teaching model. What are we missing? What else could be done for this patient? Should we move this patient to a more acute service? Are there tests results we failed to address or additional tests that should be ordered? All of this would need to be tested in a pragmatic trial. Since many hospitals have a reactive rapid response team that is called after a patient shows signs of a rapid demise, these same teams could use the probability of unexpected death to proactively round on patients before the demise. By using AI tools, hospitals can move from lagging to leading indicators.

Autopsy information on the patients who die unexpectedly could create a feedback loop for a continuous quality improvement project. This information may contribute to new knowledge in the unexpected death research and at the morbidity and mortality conferences.[5] One of the drivers of the U.S. News and World Report ranking is the observed to expected mortality. Use of AI to predict and prevent unexpected deaths is likely to be key here, but the implementation must be perfected until the outcomes are improved in a rigorous adaptive platform randomized controlled trial (RCT). Putting a spin on the results or hyping AI will not result in better outcome or better rankings. If the results are negative, accept the findings and try another implementation.

> *The whole of science is nothing more than a refinement of everyday thinking.*
>
> —ALBERT EINSTEIN.

As explained throughout the book, our approach is to create a model that is based on data from the first 24 hours for the patient's hospital admission and then compute an admission probability of a complication, like a pressure injury for example. This probability remains displayed in the EHR during the hospital stay. A second probability is created based on the most recent data. We use the same predictors and the same weights each day. Some will argue that you need to make the modeling process on a daily basis. A better approach is to use the model created from the data within the first 24 hours and then update it with new data for that patient each day, and other areas of medicine take the same approach. Perfectionist will try to obtain a new data set from day 2 and use different factors and different weights. This type of complexity slows forward progress. Perfectionist can become paralyzed and fail to make any progress.

> *"In times of change, learners inherit the Earth; while the learned find themselves beautifully equipped to deal with a world that no longer exists."*
>
> —ERIC HOFFER, AMERICAN PHILOSOPHER.

Don't we want to strive for a perfect model? What do we use as a gauge? How do we know when we are crossing over into perfectionistic thinking? The answer to these questions lies in the pragmatic results you are achieving with patient outcomes.

Understand the difference between decimal dust and scientific rigor

> *"Some AI researchers brag about how many leading zeros they have in their P value—just to show they have a sense of humor."*

A P value of $P = .00000000000000000171$ is not as important as the 95% confidence intervals around an important metric.

Your AI tool should be as precise and accurate as you can make it, but it must also be something that can be implemented in practice. The effector arm must be as strong as possible, but it must also be something that can be incorporated into a busy clinical workflow. This is the sweet spot.

> *"All models are wrong, but some are useful."*
>
> —GEORGE E. P. BOX.

Predictive models are never perfect but are generally much better than humans (Figure 8.1). The big question is whether an imperfect model can be used to focus interventions and prevention. Suppose all the patients in the hospital have a probability of some outcome and are sorted from highest down to the lowest. If the high-risk patients bubble up to the top of the list and receive the prevention resources that they need, it does not matter whether their probability of the outcomes was 92.1% or 94.3%. In effect, the implementation treats the probability like a rank. Therefore, it is more important to focus on implementing an RCT than spending years improving the AUC. When interpreting an ROC and calibration curve, it is important to consider the clinical meaning of the risk. The model may be unable to distinguish between very, very high risk, and very, very, very high risk, but this often does not matter. Furthermore, for rare conditions, there will never be sufficient data to make to upper tail of the calibration curve perfect.

> *Striving for* excellence *motivates you; striving for* perfection *is* demoralizing.
>
> —HARRIET BERYL BRAIKER.

PRINCIPLE 106 • Predictive analytics can be used to find positive deviants in the data. These data represent a departure from the norm—in a positive way.

> *"The most exciting phrase in science is not 'Eureka!' but 'That's odd!'"*
>
> —DAVID COX AND ISAAC ASIMOV.

Among patients with a very high probability of having an in-hospital complication, based on a model, some will not develop the complication. Studying these patients can often be very informative.[6] Who was predicted to be readmitted but was not? Why not? What can we learn about their resilience? What can we learn about how to improve the model? This information can teach how to improve patient outcomes and how to improve the model. Was there a treatment that these patients received that prevented the predicted outcome from happening? Does the model perform poorly in a subgroup? Some of this can be learned from chart review and some can be learned from statistical analyses.

Lessons learned from building hospital readmission predictive models

Everyone knows that hospital readmissions are a major problem in our health care system but what is less well known is that in a systematic review of the many approaches to fix this problem, Hansen et al[3] showed that nothing worked for the prevention of readmissions—unless the intervention was combined with risk stratification and focused on the patients at highest risk of readmissions. Humans cannot predict hospital complications better than a predictive model. In nearly all cases, a computerized predictive model is not only faster and cheaper but also more accurate and precise. Some clinicians will claim that they can predict which patients will be readmitted to the hospital, but when tested, they do not do much better than flipping a coin (see Figure 8.1).[7]

When we first began building a predictive model of hospital readmissions, we asked the experts to list the predictors that should be considered for the model. The first expert told us with great confidence that the best predictor was a lack of health insurance. Notice, people will often substitute an easier question that they can answer, rather than answer the question asked.

> *"This is the essence of intuitive heuristics: when faced with a difficult question, we often answer an easier one instead, usually without noticing the substitution."*
> —DANIEL KAHNEMAN, 2002 NOBEL LAUREATE.[8]

The first question is "Which variable will be the best predictor of a 30-day readmission?" The second (easier, substitution) question is "What do I remember about the most recent patient that I had who was readmitted?" When we analyzed the data on more than 100,000 patients, not only was lack of insurance not a predictor, but the exact opposite was true. Patients with the best insurance have the highest readmission rates. Clinicians, like all humans, often have predictable systematic errors in thinking, or biases, in judgments assessing risk. AI can provide clinical decision support to reduce these errors.

After we built our predictive model of hospital readmissions, some suggested that the model was incomplete or used the wrong predictors and would be benefitted by using psychosocial factors as the predictors. When we tested these, however, not only did they not improve the model, but the direction was the opposite of what was proposed—and this was statistically significant. People with the highest literacy had the highest readmission rates. The bottom line is that the clinical and laboratory data allowed us to predict hospital readmissions, while social determinants of health did not improve the model. Furthermore, laboratory predictors measure medical issues and avoid some of the ethical issues of including social determinants of health.

A predictive "impactibility" model can be used to identify a subset of patients at risk of readmission who are most likely to be impacted by preventive care. Among all of the patients predicted to be readmitted, there may be a subset that will benefit more and be amenable to preventive care. This needs to be studied for effectiveness and fairness.

> "*[There is] a puzzling limitation of our mind: our excessive confidence in what we believe we know, and our apparent inability to acknowledge the full extent of our ignorance, and the uncertainty of the world we live in. We are prone to overestimate how much we understand about the world ….*"

—DANIEL KAHNEMAN, 2002 NOBEL LAUREATE.[8]

From Kahneman, D. *Thinking, Fast and Slow.* Farrar, Straus and Giroux, 2011.

PRINCIPLE 107 • Sepsis is the 11th leading cause of death in this country and AI can give doctors the lead time they need for prevention and treatment.

In a reactive system, lagging indicators alert clinicians to the fact that a patient already has a health condition, such as sepsis. In a system that uses data to predict and prevent, leading indicators alert clinicians to the probability that a patient will develop a condition such as sepsis in the near future. A successful health care system must change from a reactive organization that uses lagging indicators to a proactive organization that uses modern sophisticated AI-based leading indicators that are evidence based.

Some research suggests that a model that can predict sepsis earlier than a physician can increase the survival rate. So, the experiment needs to measure the time to diagnosis for the model vs usual care. A logistic regression model can predict sepsis on admission to the hospital and then be updated every day with factors such as arterial blood gases measured, C-reactive protein, pneumonia, lactate, red cell distribution width, sodium, bicarbonate, albumin, Braden scale, cancer patient, base excess, surgical patient, a hospital transfer patient, oxygen saturation, pressure injury, blood pressure, carbon dioxide, arterial oxygen pressure, gender, hemoglobin, mean corpuscular hemoglobin concentration, white blood cell count, major diagnostic categories (diabetes, chronic obstructive pulmonary disease, HIV, etc), age, and vital signs.

ℹ FOR MORE INFORMATION

U.S. News & World Report. FAQ: How and Why We Rank and Rate Hospitals.[9]

CHAPTER SUMMARY

Demonstrating outcome improvement beyond that of usual care is contingent upon merging AI prediction with implementation. Strong leadership, excellent teamwork, and new incentives are needed to overcome the many hurdles.

REFERENCES

1. Warner JL, Zhang P, Liu J, Alterovitz G. Classification of hospital acquired complications using temporal clinical information from a large electronic health record. *J Biomed Inf.* 2016;59:209-217.
2. Young EW. Avoiding preventable complications in hospitalized patients with CKD. *Clin J Am Soc Nephrol.* 2017;12(5):713-714.
3. Hansen LO, Young RS, Hinami K, Leung A, Williams MV. Interventions to reduce 30-day rehospitalization: a systematic review. *Ann Intern Med.* 2011;155(8):520-528.
4. Lundberg SM, Nair B, Vavilala MS, et al. Explainable machine-learning predictions for the prevention of hypoxaemia during surgery. *Nat Biomed Eng.* 2018;2(10):749-760.
5. Lundberg GD. *Severed Trust: Why American Medicine Hasn't Been Fixed.* Basic Books; 2001.
6. Bhatt J, Zanetti C. *Big Data with a Personal Touch: The Convergence of Predictive Analytics and Positive Deviance.* The Huffington Post. 2014. Retrieved 2015-08-31. https://www.huffpost.com/entry/big-data-with-a-personal_b_5209857
7. Allaudeen N, Schnipper JL, Orav EJ, Wachter RM, Vidyarthi AR. Inability of providers to predict unplanned readmissions. *J Gen Intern Med.* 2011;26(7):771-776.
8. Kahneman D. *Thinking, Fast and Slow.* Farrar, Straus and Giroux; 2011.
9. US News & World Report. FAQ: how and why we rank and rate hospitals. https://health.usnews.com/health-care/best-hospitals/articles/faq-how-and-why-we-rank-and-rate-hospitals

13

Prevention—
Identifying Diseases
With Predictive
Models

Predictive models are more likely to be implemented and have an impact when they are truly practical. Therefore, to build practical models, the predictors should be evaluated in a logical order starting from the left as given in Table 13.1 and moving to the right. If a model focuses on genetic data or biomarkers but fail to incorporate the variables in the left columns of the table, such as body mass index (BMI), they will not be useful for real-time predictive modeling projects.

PRINCIPLE 108 • Be "Upstreamist" by using AI tools to improve prevention.

Our current health care system catches too many medical problems "downstream" after a silent period and too often in a reactive way. Obviously, there are a myriad of factors that influence this, but it is not unreasonable to think that many health conditions can be predicted earlier with AI predictive models. For example, as patients are seen for minor ailments, elective procedures, and annual checkups, the AI system could identify patients with undiagnosed and very treatable conditions such as hemochromatosis. This not only improves patient outcomes but could secondarily increase revenue for the health care system in an ethical way. Even a very thorough annual physical examination fails to catch many problems as early as AI tools could. In addition to "upstreamist" approaches in traditional health care settings, AI can also be used to predict and prevent many sports injuries and this is an area with great potential.

PRINCIPLE 109 • Measure and record how upstream conditions are diagnosed and treated in the EHR.

As said throughout this book, too much focus has been on improving the area under the receiver-operating-characteristic curve of new models. Although

TABLE 13.1	Categories of Potential Predictors Sorted by Their "Cost" and Availability			
Free by Asking	**Almost Free**	**Low Cost**	**High Cost**	**High Cost and Experimental**
Age	Blood pressure	CBC	Genetics	Biomarkers
Height	Temperature	BMP	GWAS	Liquid biopsy
Weight	O_2 saturation	CMP	Blood gases	NLP
Body mass index	Pulse	ECG	fMRI	
Sex/Gender		Retinal scan		
Smoking status		RDW		
Exercise level		WBC		
Level of stress		BUN		
Medications		Chloride		

BMP, basic metabolic panel; BUN, blood urea nitrogen; CBC, complete blood count; CMP, comprehensive metabolic panel; ECG, electrocardiogram; fMRI, functional magnetic resonance imaging; GWAS, *genome-wide association study;* NLP, natural language processing; RDW, red cell distribution width; WBC, white blood cell count

the precision of the model is very important, additional attention should be placed on moving the models into care and testing. For example, models do not need to be more precise for readmissions or sepsis; they need to be displayed to the care team earlier in the hospitalization so that the care team can act on this information. Therefore, "time to initial diagnosis" needs to be measured and recorded in a consistent way for each condition.

> *"The last mile of clinical implementation thus ends up being the far more critical task of predicting events early enough for a relevant intervention to influence care decisions and outcomes."*
>
> —JONATHAN CHEN.[1]

PRINCIPLE 110 • Health care funding of AI projects needs to prioritize prevention and wellness programs.

Across the nation, employee wellness programs have been created for many reasons and most have experienced use and positive reception. Prediction is applicable here as well, and in addition to prediction, AI tools can also add value with counterfactual "What if?" calculators (Figure 13.1).

> *"The absence of disease is not health."*
> —SHAWN ACHOR.

PRINCIPLE 111 • AI tools that display probabilities based on rigorous evidence will replace outdated rule-based systems.

Wellness programs often include a health risk assessment (HRA), which generates a report with an overall wellness score. Sometimes there are simplistic risk warnings, but this is often based on arbitrary rules (BMI > 30, age > 40, etc) and could be greatly improved by using more precise predictive models; for example, the following factors can be used to identify people at high risk for developing type 2 diabetes: age, gender, BMI (height and weight), family history of diabetes, blood pressure, race, and exercise level.

There are public websites that provide education, resources, and a risk assessment, such as https://doihaveprediabetes.org/. These are wonderful resources aimed at improving the public's overall health. These algorithms would be improved by using more modern methods, for example, age and weight should not be categorized, and blood pressure and exercise should not be dichotomized. The outcome should not be on a scale of 0 to 10, instead it would be better as a meaningful probability from 0% to 100%. These models can be improved with more laboratory data, such as cholesterol. It would be advantageous for patients to embed models into electronic health records so that they are automated as part of routine care. With the addition of an effector arm, such as a referral to the national diabetes prevention program, patients would be empowered to change.

PRINCIPLE 112 • The "paradox of prevention" states that for some health conditions, investing funding in those at low risk has a better return on investment.

According to some estimates, up to 70% of chronic disease is attributable to behavioral factors, which makes a case for the implementation of wellness

Timeframe (select one)				Hypothetical Probabilities										
[ ] 1 year, [ ] 5 years, [X] 10 years					Cancer	Heart disease	Alzheimer's	Stroke	Diabetes	Heart Attack	Hypertension	Hypercholesteremia	Lung disease	Obesity	Death
			Now		21%	33%	1%	13%	40%	10%	100%	100%	13%	100%	5%
				What if?	12%	5%	1%	5%	15%	5%	70%	80%	5%	80%	1%
Daily modifiable behaviors	Low-fat diet	1	4												
	Exercise days/week	0	5												
	Smoking status	1	0												
	Seat belt	1	1												
	Breakfast	1	1												
	Snacking	3	2												
	Strength exercise	0	3												
	Fruits and vegetables	2	3												
Long-term modifiable factors	BMI	29.1	25												
	Cholesterol	235	199												
	BP (systolic)	135	120												
	BP (diastolic)	90	80												
Nonmodifiable factors	Age	45	45												
	Gender (0-female, 1-male)	1	1												

FIGURE 13.1. Using predictive models as a "What-if?" behavioral intervention. These hypothetical values are used to show vaporware of how predictive models could be used to motivate patients to improve their daily health behaviors. By showing the probabilities of future health outcomes with the current lifestyle and contrasting that to the possible outcomes with improved lifestyle, the predictive models could be used as a motivational tool.

programs. An enormous amount of money has been invested in prevention measures that seek to lower the risk level of people at high risk for chronic disease, such as obese smokers. Research has shown that this is rarely successful, and even when it is, these individuals do not return to the same level of health as the low-risk individuals, and this did not positively affect health care costs.[2] A more successful approach may be to focus prevention on those at low risk by implementing AI tools to identify them at an early stage before they move into a higher risk category. For example, among those with a normal BMI, predict who is likely to become obese and focus on lifestyle modification. Predicting and preventing in this way is more likely to be beneficial.

The relative importance of genetics for predictive models for the development of chronic disease needs more research. To date, predictive models rarely show that genetic information alone contributes a significant amount in the prediction of some of the most common chronic health conditions. For example, type 2 diabetes is almost completely preventable and reversible with two healthy behaviors, exercise and maintaining a normal BMI.[3] Genetics, while influential, plays a smaller role in this. Research has found that the modifiable lifestyle behaviors that should be targeted in health promotion programs include low-fat diet, aerobic exercise, nonsmoking, and adequate sleep.[4]

> **ℹ️ FOR MORE INFORMATION**
>
> Modifiable Healthy Lifestyle Behaviors: 10-Year Health Outcomes From a Health Promotion Program (Daniel Byrne et al).[4]

> **CHAPTER SUMMARY**
>
> AI risk tools can be used to move health care prevention upstream. This will require new metrics for quantifying how early conditions are diagnosed. The increased precision that AI will provide will enable many prevention efforts to be more cost-effective.

REFERENCES

1. Chen JH, Asch SM. Machine learning and prediction in medicine—beyond the peak of inflated expectations. *N Engl J Med.* 2017;376(26):2507-2509.
2. Goetzel RZ, Henke RM, Head MA, Benevent R, Rhee K. Ten modifiable health risk factors and employees' medical costs-an update. *Am J Health Promot.* 2020;34(5):490-499.

3. Rolando L, Byrne DW, McGown PW, Goetzel RZ, Elasy TA, Yarbrough MI. Health risk factor modification predicts incidence of diabetes in an employee population: results of an 8-year longitudinal cohort study. *J Occup Environ Med.* 2013;55(4):410-415.

4. Byrne DW, Rolando LA, Aliyu MH, et al. Modifiable healthy lifestyle behaviors: 10-year health outcomes from a health promotion program. *Am J Prev Med.* 2016;51(6):1027-1037.

CHAPTER 14

Precision Medicine—AI to Improve Health Screenings and Treatments

Precision medicine seeks to identify health care approaches based on genetics, environment, lifestyle, and laboratory results. Artificial Intelligence (AI) is needed to integrate this information into an actionable form.

PRINCIPLE 113 • Precision screening is needed before we will have precision medicine.

AI can help nonspecialists screen their patients with the expertise of a specialist.[1] This will be an important application of AI in areas with a shortage of specialists. Health care needs to move beyond the current methods of deciding who needs screening to an AI method that is evidence based and provides probabilities (Table 14.1). Only 55% of Americans receive the recommended health care.[2]

PRINCIPLE 114 • For patients with rare conditions or confusing symptoms, AI tools are used to mine large data sets to find other similar patients and provide clues for faster diagnosis and optimal treatment.

Patients with rare, or difficult to diagnose, conditions often have a long and frustrating experience seeking opinions from doctor to doctor until their disease is diagnosed. Predictive models can shorten a patient's diagnostic odyssey, but these need to be implemented into routine care.

TABLE 14.1	Advantages of Moving From Scoring Systems to an AI Probability Model

Scoring System	AI Model
Manual	Automated
Crude	Precise and accurate
High heterogeneity	Low heterogeneity
Clinician burnout	Give clinicians time to spend with patients
Poor use of resources	Focuses limited prevention resources

Precision medicine models can reduce overtreatment

Use AI tools to be smarter at matching primary prevention to the people who will benefit the most and have the least risk of harm. AI will provide more precision in helping to decide which patients need surgery, for example, for removal of a thyroid tumor. Many patients undergo unnecessary procedures, for example, thyroid gland excision and then a lifetime of treatment. AI tools can identify which suspicious thyroid growths are cancerous and need to be removed.

PRINCIPLE 115 • AI has great potential to help change patient behavior, but the implementation and evaluations remain challenging.

Much of the development and outcomes related to chronic diseases are caused by behaviors that patients can control. These include eating a healthy low-fat diet, exercising, not smoking, moderate alcohol consumption, sleeping, and medication adherence. Much of the research on AI tools in this area has been weak and short term. Success requires long-term assessment of outcomes and rigorous scientific evaluations. The skills required to change patient behaviors are very different from the skills required to build a model. The multidisciplinary team needs to tackle these problems together.

AI tools are needed to improve the percent of patients who fill and properly adhere to the full course of a prescription treatment. Models can be used to identify those most likely to quit smoking and invest in the prevention program for them. Models can be used to enroll people who are more likely to benefit from a diabetes prevention program.[3]

PRINCIPLE 116 • **Precision medicine tools are being created and published at a rapid pace, but there is a need to test and, if they improve outcomes, implement in routine care.**

Below are examples from a wide range of medical fields illustrating how AI screening tools could play an important role in future health care (Table 14.2).

TABLE 14.2	**Opportunities for Implementing AI Screening Tools**

Health Conditions
Hypercholesterolemia
Hypertension
Cancer
    Mammogram
    Pap test
    Colonoscopy
    Computed tomography screening for lung cancer
Heart disease
Stroke
Depression
Type 2 diabetes
Hepatitis C

Health Care Utilization
Emergency department visit
Hospitalization
High health care costs
Need for a primary care physician annual exam
Need for mental health counseling

Workplace Factors
Workplace injury
Absenteeism
Presenteeism
Retention/turnover
Disability injury

1. **Prostate Cancer.**

The current approach to detecting men at early stages with prostate cancer does not use the existing data in the smartest way to optimize health outcomes. A predictive model that automatically computes the risk of not just prostate cancer but also cancer that will result in metastatic disease, poor quality of life, and death is needed. The models should include the prostate-specific antigen, age, family history of prostate cancer, prior biopsy, and result of a digital rectal exam. Nomograms are available, but these are outdated, manual, and weak. Online calculators are available, but the models need to be automated and integrated into the electronic health record and workflow (https://riskcalc.org/PCPTRC/). Biomarkers and genetic information may be useful to add to the model in the future, but this needs to be tested. A wide range of factors need to be assessed to improve these models (see Tables 6.4 and 6.5).

2. **Hemochromatosis.**

Models can detect undiagnosed diseases to help with the "If I had only known sooner" problem.

An excellent example of how AI could be used to improve health outcomes is with the early detection of hereditary hemochromatosis, which is present in about 1 in every 300 individuals in the United States. This is a common genetic disorder in which the body absorbs an excess of iron. Although the condition is present at birth, it is often symptomless until late in life when it is too late to treat effectively. In our current reactive health care system without AI, patients are not diagnosed until they are 48 years of age on average.[4] With an AI predictive model, these patients could be identified early in life (with a genetic test) and instructed to donate blood every few months to reduce their iron levels. By doing so, they could lead a normal, healthy life rather than suffering the poor outcome that is common now. Without this early detection, patients often suffer from liver cancer, cirrhosis, heart disease, arthritis, and diabetes. The AI model would provide a probability of hemochromatosis and those with the highest risk would be referred to a hematologist who would evaluate the need for the definitive genetic test. To assess if this AI approach improves health outcomes, patients would be randomized to usual care vs the AI model with the hematologist/genetic testing. The short-term end point would be age at diagnosis of hemochromatosis. The long-term end points would be age at death and quality of life. A simple logistic regression model can be created from age and other factors gathered from an annual physical, such as red cell distribution width, hematocrit, mean corpuscular hemoglobin concentration, creatinine, race, cancer, and congestive heart failure.

3. **Brown recluse spider bites.**

A brown recluse spider bite can go unnoticed by many—but for some it is lethal. A model comparing these groups not only explains why, but provides a tool that could be used to compute the probability of poor outcomes for patients seen in an emergency department.[5]

4. **Multiple myeloma.**

Multiple myeloma is a type of cancer that is often slow to be diagnosed, and then treatments can be less effective, but if diagnosed earlier, the prognosis is much better. Since this is a blood disorder, AI predictive models can compute the probability of multiple myeloma from routine blood tests in an annual physical. A model can be created using the following variables: hematocrit, CO_2, albumin, platelet count, age, blood urea nitrogen, hemoglobin, potassium, red cell distribution width, reticulocyte count, white blood cell count, sex, bodily pain (back, chest, rib), nosebleed, mean corpuscular volume, calcium, recent fracture, and erythrocyte sedimentation rate. This model could be assessed to determine whether the disease can be caught at an earlier stage and would lead to improved health outcomes. AI can also be used to reverse engineer which patients with multiple myeloma benefited from stem cell transplants so that this information could be used going forward for other patients.

5. **Colonoscopy.**

Colonoscopy screening is expensive and the criteria for screening are overly simplistic (age $\geq$ 45). AI could reduce costs and improve outcomes with models for the probability of needing a colonoscopy, not getting a colonoscopy, developing colon cancer, dying from colon cancer, and developing Lynch syndrome.

6. **Mental health screening.**

In many areas, there is a shortage of mental health professionals. For many conditions, like clinical depression, the idea of one-size-fits-all is outdated. AI can identify subtypes of depression and help identify the treatment that works best for that subtype.

Many large organizations are looking for ways to screen people at risk for suicide. One method is to survey individuals asking a series of mental health screening questions and compute probability of suicide. The respondents can be rank ordered so that those most at risk receive the prevention services that they need. Screening for suicide can be performed in tiers with branching logic. Tier 1 would ask a few basic questions. Tier 2 would ask more specific questions. Tier 3 would identify the probability of suicide. This approach will avoid asking most people questions that are not important for them to answer. Colin Walsh at Vanderbilt has been doing some excellent work in the area of real-time predictive models of suicide attempt risk.[6]

7. **Lung cancer.**
Use a real-time predictive model to select persons for lung cancer screening, rather than simplistic crude categories.

Lung cancer is one of the leading causes of cancer death and most are caught late in the disease when treatments are less effective and survival shorter. Low-dose computed tomography (CT) screening for lung cancer among current and former heavy smokers has been proven to reduce the number of deaths.[7] Unfortunately, this screening tool is not being implemented in an optimal way. AI is needed on two levels. First, to more precisely predict which patients are likely to have lung cancer and second to improve the detection of early-stage lung cancer.[8]

The criteria for screening of "current or former heaver smoker" are part of a simple approach. AI can provide a much more accurate model of who requires CT screening. Like many guidelines in medicine, the current criteria are a good starting point but can be easily improved upon with a model incorporating factors such as age, calcium, blood urea nitrogen, chronic obstructive pulmonary disease, smoking status, pack-years, years since quitting, level of education, body mass index (BMI), and family history of lung cancer. Then the probability of lung cancer can be computed as a logistic regression model: $1/(1 + 2.718^{-Z})$, with $Z = -5.839+(age - 0.045)+(predictor2 \times -0.230)....$, for example. A second deep learning model could then be used to include the CT screening data to compute probability of lung cancer.

8. **Improving end-of-life advance care planning discussions.**
AI tools can identify patients who are likely to die in the near future to ensure that the quality of their remaining life is optimal. About 25% of cancer patients have poor goals of care and therefore too many patients die in the ICU. Their last few weeks would have been improved with palliative care in hospice or at home. Although this is a sensitive subject, the hesitancy to plan creates huge financial hardships for the survivors but more important many patients spend their last few weeks in ways that are not aligned with their goals.

Our group has shown that "the optimal strategy for implementing mortality-predicting algorithms to facilitate clinical care, prognostic discussions, and palliative care interventions remains unknown." We developed and validated a predictive mortality model for adult patients from a large retrospective cohort. The model helps quantify the potential need for palliative care referrals based on risk strata.[9]

Once a patient is diagnosed with cancer or any serious disease, the big question they have is "How long will I have to live?" In our current health care system, the answer is unnecessarily vague. AI tools can provide a much more precise and accurate estimate. These can be provided along with 95% confidence intervals to provide a measure of uncertainty. Physicians typically estimate that a patient will live 3 times longer than they actually live. A predictive model of how long a patient will live can be created with routine variables, such as age, gender, red cell distribution width, blood pressure, white blood cell count, Braden scale, albumin, oxygen saturation, blood urea nitrogen, platelet count, BMI, etc.

 FOR MORE INFORMATION

MIT OpenCourseWare. Lecture 20. Precision medicine. Machine Learning for Healthcare. Peter Szolovits.[10]
PatientsLikeMe.
https://en.wikipedia.org/wiki/PatientsLikeMe.

CHAPTER SUMMARY

AI can make precision medicine a reality by providing both accuracy and precision. AI will also be used for screenings in ways that the screening device was not intended. For example, retinal scans are demonstrating value in predicting heart disease. Liquid biopsies and other general blood tests will become valuable in the near future in AI tools. Electrocardiograms combined with machine learning are providing diagnoses that cardiologists cannot identify. AI will be used to diagnose conditions and complications earlier and earlier. AI will also provide risk-benefit information for surgeons to be more evidence based about whether or not to operate on a patient. Rigorous evaluations are needed that these tools are implemented appropriately for all.

REFERENCES

1. Milea D, Najjar RP, Zhubo J, et al. Artificial intelligence to detect papilledema from ocular fundus photographs. *N Engl J Med*.2020;382(18):1687-1695.
2. McGlynn EA, Asch SM, Adams J, et al. The quality of health care delivered to adults in the United States. *N Engl J Med*. 2003;348(26):2635-2645.

3. Chakkalakal RJ, Connor LR, Rolando LA, et al. Putting the national diabetes prevention program to work: predictors of achieving weight-loss goals in an employee population. *Prev Chronic Dis*. 2019;16:E125.

4. Nowak A, Giger RS, Krayenbuehl PA. Higher age at diagnosis of hemochromatosis is the strongest predictor of the occurrence of hepatocellular carcinoma in the Swiss hemochromatosis cohort: a prospective longitudinal observational study. *Medicine (Baltim)*. 2018;97(42):e12886.

5. Loden JK, Seger DL, Spiller HA, Wang L, Byrne DW. Cutaneous-hemolytic loxoscelism following brown recluse spider envenomation: new understandings. *Clin Toxicol*. 2020;58(12):1297-1305.

6. Walsh CG, Johnson KB, Ripperger M, et al. Prospective validation of an electronic health record-based, real-time suicide risk model. *JAMA Netw Open*. 2021;4(3):e211428.

7. National Lung Screening Trial Research Team, Aberle DR, Adams AM, et al. Reduced lung-cancer mortality with low-dose computed tomographic screening. *N Engl J Med*. 2011;365(5):395-409.

8. Tammemägi MC, Katki HA, Hocking WG, et al. Selection criteria for lung-cancer screening. *N Engl J Med*. 2013;368(8):728-736. Erratum in: *N Engl J Med*. 2013;369(4):394.

9. Agarwal R, Domenico HJ, Balla SR, et al. Palliative care exposure relative to predicted risk of 6-month mortality in hospitalized adults. *J Pain Symptom Manag*. 2022; 63(5):645-653. doi:10.1016/j.jpainsymman.2022.01.013

10. Szolovits P. MIT OpenCourseWare. Lecture 20. Precision medicine. Machine Learning for Healthcare. https://www.youtube.com/watch?v=kZrb6ZIwJqg

Drugs and Devices—Using AI to Improve Pharmaceutical and Medical Device Development and Applications

PRINCIPLE 117 • **Deep learning methods are being used to efficiently solve complex problems such as predicting the three-dimensional structure of proteins.**

Since 1994, there has been a competition, known as CASP—"Critical Assessment of Structure Prediction," in which contestants compete to predict protein structures. Recently DeepMind, an Artificial Intelligence (AI) company owned by Google, applied deep learning methods to make significant advances in solving the problem of protein structure prediction. The team also published the data and open-source code for their neural network called the AlphaFold model.[1] This project is an excellent example of intelligence amplification provided by AI.

We saw that with low-dimensional data, logistic regression often produces more useful predictive models, but with high-dimensional data such as protein folding, logistic regression is the wrong tool and deep learning is needed. Yet, deep learning has data inefficiency limitations requiring massive data sets, so it is not always the best approach. The key is to use the right AI tool for a given problem.

PRINCIPLE 118 • **AI will both speed drug development and increase the approval success rate.**

The current drug development process is unsustainable—90% of drugs fail in their randomized controlled trials (RCTs). The cost to bring a new drug

197

to market is more than $1 billion. While machine learning is often used for analysis in the research phase, the analytic approach is not always implemented in the practice of drug discovery. So, researchers need to close the loop and perform validation studies of AI tools that take the findings from a research paper to the next level of drug discovery. Pharmaceutical companies and biotech startups that effectively implement AI to revamp the drug development pipeline will have the competitive advantage.

Trial and error of therapeutic molecules is transitioning to engineering molecules and drugs with specific properties for high-quality therapeutics. *In silico* AI tools are being used to improve drug dosage research, which can be a significant improvement over the current antiquated process. An AI model that computes the probability that a research participant will complete the trial could speed progress and cut costs.

PRINCIPLE 119 • Drug discovery will be hastened by a greater understanding of disease subtypes.

> *"AI will take the 'idio' out of idiopathic."*

Research often shows us that what was once thought of as one disease is actually several distinct diseases. Unsupervised learning is being used to define such disease clusters and the subclassification system for each. This is fascinating and valuable work because the noise caused by the current heterogeneity of the treatment effect has made it difficult and expensive to bring new drugs to the market. Examples of heterogeneous diseases that have better outcomes as the result of understanding the subtypes include sepsis, asthma, depression, cancer, autism, heart disease, and adult respiratory distress syndrome.

PRINCIPLE 120 • Focusing on the patients who will benefit most from a new drug will be achievable through modern risk stratification and predictive modeling.

Predictive models can help streamline clinical trials by providing risk stratification which aids in the study of drugs and devices, allowing those researchers to home in on the patients who will benefit most. This increases the odds of a successful trial and lowers costs.

Predictive enrichment refers to the use of predictive models to identify a homogeneous subtype of a disease to facilitate efficient treatment research.

The goal is to identify patients <u>most likely to respond</u> to a drug based on a biological mechanism.

Prognostic enrichment refers to the use of a model to select patients with a higher likelihood of having a disease-related outcome of interest, such as mortality. The goal is to identify patients <u>most likely to have the study end point</u>.

PRINCIPLE 121 • Side effects, adverse drug events, and drug-drug interactions can be reduced with predictive modeling.

The cost of this problem has been estimated at $3.5 billion. The current approach of starting a patient on a drug, such as a particular statin, and seeing if they develop a reaction will be replaced with an approach that uses AI tools to compute the probability of a reaction. We have previously shown that it is possible to predict adverse drug events in hospitalized patients with a predictive model.[2] Although much research has been conducted in this area, the challenge is moving it into clinical care and assessing the impact.

Genetic information can be used to determine the right dose, the right drug, at the right time, with more accuracy than usual care. But this genetic information should be combined with other nongenetic factors to build a more complete model. This precision medicine approach needs to be assessed in a large pragmatic trial with the scientists leading the project—not the marketing people. The results of such a trial need to be published in a way that other scientists can evaluate the data.

PRINCIPLE 122 • Robotics used in health care will expand and machine learning techniques have great potential for enhancing their impact.

Although robotic tools have long been used in medicine, what is new is the addition of modern machine learning methods. The principles in this book also apply to medical robotics, but some (such as randomization and intention to treat) may be new to some robotics developers. Physician-scientists will need to lead these projects to ensure that these tools are tested with rigorous science to improve patient outcomes.

The da Vinci surgical robot was approved by the Food and Drug Administration in 2000 and has been used in millions of surgeries. In general, patients benefit from smaller incisions, reduced blood loss, and faster recovery. We can expect to see medical robotics provide additional benefit with applications in prostheses (artificial limbs), disinfecting, transportation, radiation therapy, rehabilitation, medication delivery, vaccine testing, nanorobotics, and wearable devices, such as smartwatches. Integrating these systems into our health care system has great potential provided the decisions are based on evidence.

AI tools have the potential to improve prescription dosing and identify people who might benefit from pharmaceutical products.

Many patients have undiagnosed chronic conditions and would benefit from an appropriate prescription, such as a statin (Table 15.1). For one example of these see the "Do I have prediabetes?" risk test at https://doihaveprediabetes.org/

More than 100,000 Americans died of drug overdoses in the past year. AI tools can be used to prevent the next "opioid crisis." For example, an RCT has shown that compared with standard postdischarge oxycodone prescribing after cesarean birth, individualized opioid prescribing based on inpatient use reduced the number of unused oxycodone tablets.[3]

TABLE 15.1	**Top Prescription Drugs in the United States**		
Drug Name	**Total U.S. Patients**	**Brand Name**	**Primary Use**
Atorvastatin	24,493,971	Lipitor	Hypercholesterolemia
Amoxicillin	20,368,921	Amoxil, Trimox	Antibiotic
Lisinopril	19,990,170	Prinivil, Zestril	Hypertension
Levothyroxine	19,698,087	Synthroid, Levoxyl	Thyroid
Albuterol	19,085,418	Ventolin, Proventil	Breathing difficulty
Metformin	17,430,765	Glucophage, Fortamet	Diabetes
Amlodipine	16,419,181	Norvasc	Hypertension
Metoprolol	15,177,787	Lopressor, Toprol XL	Hypertension
Omeprazole	12,869,290	Losec, Prilosec	Gastroesophageal reflux disease
Losartan	11,760,646	Cozaar	Hypertension
Azithromycin	11,577,286	Zithromax, Azithrocin	Antibiotic

TABLE 15.1	*Continued*		

Drug Name	Total U.S. Patients	Brand Name	Primary Use
Prednisone	10,999,246	Deltasone, Orasone	Inflammation
Ibuprofen	10,951,995	Advil, Motrin	Pain
Hydrocodone/ Acetamin- ophen	10,409,764	Vicodin/Norco	Pain (Opioid)
Gabapentin	9,818,634	Neurontin	Seizures
Fluticasone	9,564,147	Flovent, Flonase	Breathing
Hydrochlo- rothiazide	9,358,879	Apo-Hydro, Microzide	Diuretic
Simvastatin	8,543,612	Zocor	Cholesterol
Sertraline	7,723,122	Zoloft, Lustral	Antidepressant
Montelukast	7,429,725	Singulair	Breathing
Pantoprazole	6,777,996	Protonix	Stomach Acid
Furosemide	6,640,042	Lasix, Frusemide	Diuretic
Meloxicam	6,484,210	Mobic, Metacam	Pain
Amoxicillin; Clavulanate	6,468,086	Augmentin, Clavulin	Antibiotic
Cephalexin	6,267,878	Keflex, Ceporex	Antibiotic
Rosuvastatin	6,129,254	Crestor, Rosulip	Cholesterol
Escitalopram	5,544,406	Cipralex, Lexapro	Antidepressant
Bupropion	5,520,278	Wellbutrin, Zyban	Antidepressant
Tramadol	5,496,843	Ultram, Zytram	Pain (Opioid)
Pravastatin	5,420,488	Pravachol, Selektine	Cholesterol

https://www.visualcapitalist.com/ranked-the-most-prescribed-drugs-in-the-u-s/

FOR MORE INFORMATION

DeepMind × UCL. Deep Learning Lecture Series. Introduction to Machine Learning and AI. Thore Graepel[4]

CHAPTER SUMMARY

Deep learning methods are proving valuable in the drug development world as demonstrated by the recent success of the DeepMind AlphaFold team's success in predicting protein structures. Unsupervised learning enables an understanding of subtypes of diseases that can make drug discovery cheaper and faster. By providing real-time predictive tools, drugs can be prescribed in a safer way to get the right drug, at the right dose, to the right patient, the first time. Robotics using machine learning has already had a huge impact in health care. In the future, many medical devices will be improved with an AI component. A major obstacle in drug development is that the needed team of experts often work in different divisions and there is a lack of collaborative opportunities. This will require restructuring so that a small team can effectively work together. Overcoming silos in the biotechnology world through multidepartment team development is just as critical as in the academic world.

REFERENCES

1. Jumper J, Evans R, Pritzel A, et al. Highly accurate protein structure prediction with AlphaFold. *Nature.* 2021;596(7873):583-589.
2. Johnston PE, France DJ, Byrne DW, et al. Assessment of adverse drug events among patients in a tertiary care medical center. *Am J Health Syst Pharm.* 2006;63(22):2218-2227.
3. Osmundson SS, Raymond BL, Kook BT, et al. Individualized compared with standard postdischarge oxycodone prescribing after cesarean birth: a randomized controlled trial. *Obstet Gynecol.* 2018;132(3):624-630.
4. Graepel T. DeepMind x UCL. Deep learning lecture series. Introduction to machine learning and AI. https://www.youtube.com/watch?v=7R52wiUgxZI

Medical Literature— AI and Information Overload

PRINCIPLE 123 • **Recognize what AI can and cannot do regarding the medical literature.**

> *"By far, the greatest danger of Artificial Intelligence is that people conclude too early that they understand it."*
>
> —ELIEZER YUDKOWSKY, AI THEORIST.

Artificial Intelligence (AI) is not the magic bullet solution for all problems in health care. Solving the information overload from the medical literature may be one of these areas that AI is not ready to solve yet (Table 16.1). To be able to critically interpret even one tiny area of the medical literature and draw a valid conclusion about a clinical question requires years of training and experience.

After a definitive randomized controlled trial (RCT) is published and the experts agree on the conclusion, AI models could be developed to learn to distinguish the previous papers that were right from those that were wrong. This would be a valuable research endeavor but a huge undertaking. The experts with this training could be incentivized to label papers as valid or invalid and an AI system could be trained to then predict valid papers,

TABLE 16.1	The Explosion of Medical Literature and Health Care Information Overload
>800,000	Medical research articles published each year
>5600	Medical journals
47,476	Total number of articles published in *The New England Journal of Medicine*
731	Articles published in *The New England Journal of Medicine* in 1 year

but this will require further research—and may be an impossible task. This would be similar to labeling images as a cat or dog and then training an AI system to predict in the future. But currently we do not have published papers labeled in this way.

> *"The complexity of modern medicine exceeds the capacity of the unaided expert mind."*
>
> —DAVID EDDY, AMERICAN PHYSICIAN, MATHEMATICIAN, AND HEALTHCARE ANALYST.

When AI vendors claim that their AI tool "reads the journals for you to save you time," recognize that there is no real understanding and that it is summarizing factoids from invalid studies—in conjunction with valid ones.

> *"There's no machine that in any deep sense understands why you can pull something with a string and not push it. Every normal child understands that sort of thing very well."*
>
> —MARVIN MINSKY, AI PIONEER.

PRINCIPLE 124 • Before AI can be used to summarize the medical literature, algorithms need to be developed to weigh the papers to separate those that are high quality from those that are flawed.[1]

The quality of the information sources could be weighted, which is likely to improve how AI summarizes the medical literature but is unlikely to be a complete solution (Table 16.2).

Here is an example to show the challenges of using AI to summarize the medical literature. The most common medical intervention in the hospital is IV fluid. Hundreds of papers have been published on the comparison of these fluids, so it is logical to have AI summarize these scientific studies and provide a recommendation. The two major choices are saline and balanced crystalloids (lactated Ringer's solution). If we were to have AI summarize the medical literature to ask "Which IV fluid is better for most hospitalized patients, saline or a balanced fluid?" it is unlikely to provide the correct answer. For example, Alexa will respond "Sorry I don't have an answer for that." The major reason is that most of these studies were based on observational data. Many believe that you can use observational data and make statistical adjustments to get the correct answer, but this rarely works for cause and effect of medical interventions. Most of the randomized studies were too small to detect a clinically meaningful effect or were flawed in some way. The correct answer is a balanced fluid, which was

TABLE 16.2	Factors to Weigh Before Summarizing the Medical Literature

Impact factor of the journal
Year of publication
Strength of the study design (observational to randomized controlled trial)
Sample size, power, event rate, confidence intervals
Funding source/conflicts of interest
Field (oncology, medicine, psychology, preclinical cancer studies, etc)
Forms of bias
Hill's criteria for causation
Number of times the paper was cited
Biostatistician coauthor[2]

only learned recently in two randomized controlled trials that we conducted at Vanderbilt.[3,4] AI works with facts in a data set, but for many questions, medicine does not have a set of facts—we have an active complex scientific debate.

PRINCIPLE 125 • **Regarding the medical literature, it is not that there is too much information but rather there is too much misinformation. Even the most advanced AI and NLP techniques cannot fix misinformation.**

"We need less research, better research, and research done for the right reasons."[5]

—Doug Altman, the late biostatistician.

AI natural language processing (NLP) projects in this area of using the medical literature to provide insights to physicians have failed partly because the AI experts did not understand that much of the medical journal literature is wrong.[6] Using AI to summarize it is not a simple solution.

"Half of what you'll learn in medical school will be shown to be either dead wrong or out of date within five years of your graduation; the trouble is that nobody can tell you which half—so the most important thing to learn is how to learn on your own."

—David Sackett, one of the fathers of Evidence-Based Medicine.

Enormous amounts of published medical research papers have created "big data." That does not, however, mean that AI can use it. Begley and Ellis were only able to replicate 6 of 53 landmark cancer studies.[7] The reproducibility crisis has also been documented by many others,[8-10] and since much of the literature is wrong, there is a low signal-to-noise ratio and AI does poorly with low signal-to-noise data. Additionally, the medical literature is unstructured and although NLP has made advances, they are not sufficient to handle the complexity of medical terminology and problems.

> *"It is not just about the quantity of data but the quality of data."*
> —LILY PENG, GOOGLE HEALTH.

Perhaps in the future AI will be able to harness the wealth of information in the published medical literature, but this will require a more advanced approach than what has been attempted previously. AI works well summarizing large bodies of literature when that literature is mostly facts with a high signal-to-noise ratio. That is, when most of the information is true and there are very few incorrect statements. For example, AI (or Alexa) could easily answer the question "What is the capital of New York?" because most of the published resources would list the correct answer "Albany." If half of the published resources listed it as Poughkeepsie or New York City, AI would fail. The signal-to-noise ratio is low in the medical literature, but it is high in the electronic health record, self-reported health risk assessments, and imaging devices.

When using medical research journals as a data source, AI has a hard time answering a complex question like "Does a postdischarge telephone call program reduce 30-day hospital readmissions?" We performed a rigorous randomized controlled pragmatic trial to answer this question and found that the answer is "No,"[11] but using AI to summarize the medical literature would most likely give the wrong answer. An experienced medical researcher with good statistical and study design training could review these papers and determine the correct conclusion, but it will take some time for AI to replicate or beat that level of real intelligence.

Meta-analysis has been proposed as the answer—combine the findings from many published papers and the truth will appear. Combining many flawed evaluations, however, does not provide the correct answer. In medicine there is a saying: "Meta-analysis is to analysis as meta-physics is to physics." Systematic reviews, such as Cochrane reviews, could provide the correct answer, and sometimes, they do, sometimes they do not. While it is true that meta-analysis does more than combine published papers, these methods are insufficient to overcome the problems listed in Table 16.3.

TABLE 16.3	Reasons Why Some Medical Literature is Flawed

1. Science is an active debate—not a set of facts.
2. Publication bias—studies that show a benefit are more likely to be accepted for publication by a medical journal. Journal editors avoid publishing papers that do not show that an intervention worked, partly because it lowers their journal's impact factor.
3. There is little incentive for research teams to publish about their own failure. They have been funded to implement interventions and are unlikely to write and submit a paper showing that their work does not provide value.
4. Low-impact journals rarely have paid statistical reviewers to critique the study design and analysis in detail and many of these journals have a high acceptance rate.
5. Approximately 58% of reviewers and editors admitted that they did not have the statistical skills needed to judge the medical journal manuscripts that they reviewed.[12]
6. Most of the papers published are based on weak observational evaluations rather than randomization.
7. Improper data analysis, for example, failing to use the intention-to-treat principle, which states that if people are randomized to the intervention, they are included in the analysis, even if they did not complete or receive the intervention.
8. The analysis, question, and hypothesis are not prespecified—fishing expeditions, recklessly looking for any $P < .05$ or spurious interactions.
9. The authors do not use Hill's criteria for causation and instead conflate correlation with causation.
10. The assumptions for the statistical methods were violated.
11. The studies were underpowered.
12. Outcome reporting bias—writing the paper in a way to make the trial appear positive. For example, focusing on one of many secondary end points that turned out significant by chance alone.
13. Spin—P value trending toward significance. Some investigators will report that their P value was not less than .05 but "was trending toward significance" as if they could perceive the intention and direction of a P value!
14. Confirmation bias—selectively quoting the literature and results that support the conclusion.

Understand precisely what NLP can accomplish vs the NLP propaganda

Using AI to provide useful information from the published medical literature will be much more challenging than simply applying NLP. Medicine is complex, and the facts are often hidden among statements that are not true. Consider how NLP would handle "Shakespeare used too many clichés." AI does not understand that this is a joke. It takes a human to understand the meaning, in a similar way it takes a human to critically interpret the medical literature—so far.

PRINCIPLE 126 • Focus on implementing "narrow AI" in a useful way rather than wasting time chasing the holy grail—artificial general intelligence (AGI).

AGI, or strong AI, refers to the hypothetical ability to perform any intellectual task that a human could, for example, critically interpreting the medical literature and summarizing with a valid conclusion. AGI may become a reality in the distant future, but currently only narrow or weak AI tools that are designed to solve specific problems are available for our use.

Singularity refers to AI that becomes smarter than humans and uncontrollable. Many AI researchers waste time working on creating a "docularity" in which the AI is smarter than a doctor. This effort would be better spent developing and implementing clinical decision support tools.

PRINCIPLE 127 • AI researchers should have high standards for what they publish and avoid contributing to the problems with the medical literature. Medical AI has a replication crisis and therefore publishing papers about an AI tool requires a new level of rigor.

Journals must make it easier to publish AI replication papers and academic medical centers must provide more career advancement credit for those who do. Journals could reserve space for replication papers. Funding agencies could look more favorably on grant applications that include (1) a robust replication plan, (2) an external temporal validation, and (3) a pragmatic RCT.

There are many ways that reporting of AI tools could be improved, such as the inclusion of a flowchart of the model building process and addition of a calibration curve. Provide sufficient detail that would be needed to replicate. Reviewers will be interested in the precision as well as the accuracy of your

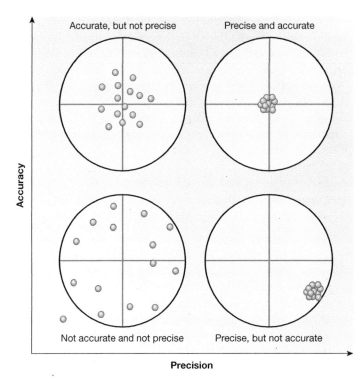

FIGURE 16.1. Precision and accuracy. AI predictive models need to be both precise and accurate.

model (Figure 16.1). If possible, put the data and code in the appendix or on github.com. The principles of reproducible research need to be applied to AI in medicine. For example, an independent biostatistician could independently reproduce the results based on what is written in the Methods and appendix of the paper before submission. More AI models need to be published in high-profile journals and following modern reporting standards will make this possible.

Therefore, plan how you will adhere to reporting standards when publishing about AI. In the Methods section of your paper, include a statement such as "reporting guidelines were followed using the Transparent Reporting of a Multivariable Prediction Model for Individual Prognosis Or Diagnosis tool.[13] The good news is that there are clear and very detailed guidelines for reporting about AI. You will need to study these before you create the model to be prepared for the writing phase. For randomized studies, follow CONSORT (consolidated standards of reporting trials). For nonrandomized studies, follow TRIPOD (Transparent Reporting of a multivariable prediction model for Individual Prognosis Or Diagnosis). Assess the risk of bias by using Cochrane risk of bias tool for randomized studies and PROBAST (prediction model risk of bias assessment tool) for nonrandomized studies. Finally, a good resource is "Minimum information about clinical artificial intelligence modeling: the MI-CLAIM checklist."[14]

The analysis plan for an AI pragmatic RCT should be prespecified in detail and documented in clinicaltrials.gov or a similar register

This should include planned interactions, interim stopping rules, model creation, model validation, etc. When results are negative, investigators will sometimes ask: Does the intervention work in any subgroup? The answer is: it will appear to work in 1/20 subgroups by chance alone with a P value $< .05$. This is not real and in the next study it will not replicate.

When the results are negative, investigators will sometimes ask: Does the intervention work in a subgroup of those with the highest baseline level of X? The answer is no, this is called regression to the mean, not evidence that the intervention works in a subgroup.

Publish a trial design paper to provide the technical and study design details and document the prespecified analysis plan. For example, this paper "Electronic health record alerts for acute kidney injury: multicenter, randomized clinical trial" published a design paper[15] and included this statement in the Methods: "A detailed description of the trial design and rationale has been previously published." For more examples, see references [16-18].

> ### ℹ️ FOR MORE INFORMATION
>
> The SPIRIT-AI and CONSORT-AI initiative—"an international collaborative effort to improve the transparency and completeness of reporting of clinical trials evaluating interventions involving artificial intelligence." SPIRIT-AI is for the protocol paper and CONSORT-AI is for the RCT.[19]
> Retraction Watch.[20]

CHAPTER SUMMARY

One can currently perform a sophisticated search of the medical literature using PubMed, Google, or Google Scholar. These can be refined to specific high-impact journals or randomized trials. The question is: Can an AI tool summarize the medical literature better than the existing search tools? Although information overload is a major problem in medicine, more work is needed before AI can summarize the medical journal literature—beyond the current search tools. The success of AI requires a mature understanding of the signal-to-noise ratio in the data source. Currently in the medical literature, this ratio is too low for our existing tools.

Medical AI has a replication crisis. Published reports need to follow modern reporting standards and focus on reproducible research. Once published, science journalists serve a vital role in communicating AI advances to the public. They must critically interpret AI evidence and avoid printing a version of a press release or the conclusion from a low-impact journal.

REFERENCES

1. Jager LR, Leek JT. An estimate of the science-wise false discovery rate and application to the top medical literature. *Biostatistics*. 2014;15(1):1-12.
2. Altman DG, Goodman SN, Schroter S. How statistical expertise is used in medical research. *JAMA*. 2002;287(21):2817-2820.
3. Semler MW, Self WH, Wanderer JP, et al. Balanced crystalloids versus saline in critically ill adults. *N Engl J Med*. 2018;378(9):829-839.
4. Self WH, Semler MW, Wanderer JP, et al. Balanced crystalloids versus saline in noncritically ill adults. *N Engl J Med*. 2018;378(9):819-828.
5. Altman DG. The scandal of poor medical research. *BMJ*. 1994;308:283.
6. Ioannidis JP. Why most published research findings are false. *PLoS Med*. 2005;2(8):e124.
7. Begley CG, Ellis LM. Drug development: raise standards for preclinical cancer research. *Nature*. 2012;483(7391):531-533.
8. Unreliable research. Trouble at the lab. *Economist*. October 19, 2013.
9. Maxwell SE, Lau MY, Howard GS. Is psychology suffering from a replication crisis? What does "failure to replicate" really mean? *Am Psychol*. 2015;70(6):487-498.
10. Allison DB, Brown AW, George BJ, Kaiser KA. Reproducibility: a tragedy of errors. *Nature*. 2016;530(7588):27-29.
11. Yiadom MYAB, Domenico HJ, Byrne DW, et al. Impact of a follow-up telephone call program on 30-day readmissions (FUTR-30): a pragmatic randomized controlled real-world effectiveness trial. *Med Care*. 2020;58(9):785-792.

12. Byrne. *Publishing Your Medical Research*. Wolters Kluwer; 2017. https://www.slideshare.net/DanielByrne12/publishing-your-medical-research-125452257

13. Collins GS, Reitsma JB, Altman DG, et al. Transparent reporting of a multivariable prediction model for Individual Prognosis or Diagnosis (TRIPOD). *Circulation*. 2015;131:211-219.

14. Norgeot B, Quer G, Beaulieu-Jones BK, et al. Minimum information about clinical artificial intelligence modeling: the MI-CLAIM checklist. *Nat Med*. 2020;26(9):1320-1324.

15. Wilson FP, Martin M, Yamamoto Y, et al. Electronic health record alerts for acute kidney injury: multicenter, randomized clinical trial. *BMJ*. 2021;372:m4786.

16. Semler MW, Self WH, Wang L, et al. Balanced crystalloids versus saline in the intensive care unit: study protocol for a cluster-randomized, multiple-crossover trial. *Trials*. 2017;18(1):129.

17. Walker SC, Creech CB, Domenico HJ, French B, Byrne DW, Wheeler AP. A real-time risk-prediction model for pediatric venous thromboembolic events. *Pediatrics*. 2021;147(6):e2020042325.

18. Yiadom MYAB, Domenico H, Byrne D, et al. Randomised controlled pragmatic clinical trial evaluating the effectiveness of a discharge follow-up phone call on 30-day hospital readmissions: balancing pragmatic and explanatory design considerations. *BMJ Open*. 2018;8(2):e019600.

19. Liu X, Rivera SC, Moher D, Calvert MJ, Denniston AK, SPIRIT-AI and CONSORT-AI Working Group. Reporting guidelines for clinical trial reports for interventions involving artificial intelligence: the CONSORT-AI extension. *BMJ*. 2020;370:m3164. The SPIRIT-AI and CONSORT-AI initiative. https://www.bmj.com/content/bmj/370/bmj.m3164.full.pdf

20. Retraction Watch. https://retractionwatch.com/

Imaging—Medical Imaging and Strategies for Assessing Patient Impact

Remarkable advances have been made in medical imaging technology, and today, there is a new layer of Artificial Intelligence (AI) being implemented on top of that technology. But as in other areas of medicine we have not seen evidence that patient outcomes are improved by adding AI to imaging. What is the stumbling block?

> *"One of the most consistent findings from clinical and health services research is the failure to translate research into practice and policy."*
>
> —JEREMY GRIMSHAW ET AL[1]

The reporting of AI imaging research and the research itself needs more real-world clinical setting studies, projects that provide access to the datasets and code, and studies that honestly report limitations and state that further prospective studies or trials are required. This requires a multidisciplinary research team that is willing to conduct an experiment that might show that their tool did not improve health outcomes—at least with the first iteration. A scientific approach may identify that the tool is not as accurate—who will fund this study? There is little incentive for the sponsor to take this on.

Here are a few facts to illustrate the importance of rigorous AI imaging research:

- It is estimated that there are 12 million diagnostic errors per year in the United States.[2]
- 10% of deaths in the hospital are attributable to diagnostic errors.
- 40,000 patients/year have a stroke missed in the emergency department.

PRINCIPLE 128 • AI imaging tools require rigorous prospective testing. Unproven AI tools should not be widely implemented in clinical practice.

When medical specialists interpret medical images, the inter-rater reliability (how well they agree with other experts) is often low and the variability of conclusions is high. This has been shown in ophthalmology,[3] radiology,[4] and pathology.[5] Their intra-rater reliability (how well they agree with themselves on the same image in the future) is not much better.[6]

So, AI should assist this field, yet while an imaging AI system can appear to perform as well as a radiologist, when tested in an alternative environment, say at another hospital, it can perform poorly. Yet if a radiologist changes jobs and moves from one hospital to another, it is very unlikely that their performance as a radiologist will fluctuate. This can be a marker of overfitting, reverse causation (label leakage), or general brittleness. Brittle AI systems need to be improved until they are more like robust radiologists by building a model carefully to avoid including inappropriate predictors (reverse causation) and performing rigorous external and geographical validations.

As discussed earlier, overfitting describes the statistical phenomenon in which a model fits the training data closer than is appropriate rather than describing the reality of the clinical relationship. An overfit model may appear to have good performance, but it is customized to the training data set so closely and will not perform as well in the future on other data sets—the external temporal validation set.

Another example of overfitting and choosing the incorrect variables/features occurred in attempts to predict tuberculosis. The chest X-rays for the model's patients who were diagnosed with tuberculosis were obtained from one hospital, while the patients without tuberculosis had X-rays from another hospital. The algorithm discriminated between the equipment and processes used at the two sites rather than between those with and without tuberculosis.

> *"Randomized controlled trials in which individual patients are randomized to receive care with a diagnostic or predictive artificial intelligence tool under investigation or care without the tool represent the strongest methodologic design for studying the value and effect of the artificial intelligence techniques."*
>
> —SEONG HO PARK ET AL[7]

PRINCIPLE 129 • Medical images are high-dimensional data problems, that is, many predictors (pixels) which require testing with neural networks and deep learning approaches.

As discussed throughout the book, deep learning and logistic regression are simply tools to solve different problems and neither is better than the other. Each has strengths and weaknesses, but deep learning has major advantages over logistic for imaging analysis. Due to the number of predictors/features (pixels) and complexity of an image, deep learning is preferred because the complexity of the data would cause numerous problems for logistic.

For predicting binary outcomes with low-dimensional data (not images), logistic regression often does as well as or better than deep learning and has the advantage of being easily coded and displayed in the electronic health record allowing the user to see what drives the probability. Deep learning suffers from black box issues, but additional user interface tools are available to overcome this concern. For many projects and papers, the best approach is to run various models and compare the performance. Again, understanding the pros and cons of using various AI tools is an important and rare skill. Related to this is the skill of knowing exactly what the various model approaches do well vs the hype about what they do well.

A myth that is often repeated to the general public is that AI tools are continuously learning from the data

This is rarely true. Models are typically developed, tested, and implemented. Until the next version of the model is implemented to replace the previous one, no changes in the algorithm occur. For many medical devices, the Food and Drug Administration (FDA) requires approval for a new version of the model and does not allow an approved model to continuously learn in clinical care. The FDA uses the following terminology: "Software developers can use machine learning to create an algorithm that is '<u>locked</u>' so that its function does not change, or '<u>adaptive</u>' so its behavior can change over time based on new data." Most AI models that involve humans are locked because it is safer to implement and monitor. Adaptive models are challenging to safely implement and require much more research. Note: this type of adaptive machine learning model is completely different from an adaptive platform trial (APT). With the APT, the implementation interventions are changed, but the AI model is not learning and changing over time, with the exception of new versions of a model.

PRINCIPLE 130 • **Published research on imaging AI must adhere to modern reporting standards and limit conclusions to the results reported.**

> *"Few prospective deep learning studies and randomised trials exist in medical imaging. Most non-randomised trials are not prospective, are at high risk of bias, and deviate from existing reporting standards."*

—MYURA NAGENDRAN ET AL[8]

PRINCIPLE 131 • *High-stakes decisions need trust.* **Explainable AI tools, such as bounding boxes, can help solve the black box problem for AI in medical imaging.**

Providing the clinician with a probability of a diagnosis from a medical image that is based on a black box remains a challenge. The probability must be accompanied with tools that explain the decision.

"Explainable" refers to the general set of techniques that aim to unveil the inner workings of the AI model on a task (eg, a dot plot of the strength of predictors). "Interpretable" refers to explanations represented in a human-readable format (eg, a heatmap). Most AI imaging tools are by their very nature a black box; it is difficult to say exactly what elements of an image are driving the prediction. This lack of "explainability" can be an obstacle to clinical acceptance. <u>Global explainability</u> refers to demonstrating how the whole model works on a large group of patients. <u>Local explainability</u> refers to demonstrating how the model is making a decision for this particular patient. Global methods include the following: (1) Classification And Regression Trees (CART), (2) SHapley Additive exPlanation (SHAP), (3) Black Box Explainable through Transparent Approximations, and (4) Local Interpretable Model-agnostic Explanations. SHAP plots are a global method of making a black box machine learning model more interpretable by showing the most influential predictors and with SHAP values quantify how the prediction of the model changes when each predictor is removed.

Black box problems have been addressed by creating CART (tree-based diagrams) showing how the inputs are related to the outcome. CART is not a good option for creating or explaining a high-dimensional model, but it is a good option for displaying a low-dimensional model. CART is also useful for detective work to understand the missing data, interactions, and understanding subgroups, for example, how a model performs differently for men and women.

Local, patient-specific methods are generally based on a box or heatmap superimposed on the image, that is the "Show me where" bounding box. An attention heatmap will show the radiologist the specific part of an image, for example, a mammogram that caused it to compute a high probability of breast cancer. The clinician may see what is causing the prediction and realize that it is a meaningless artifact or may look closer and see something that was missed. This could also be a valuable teaching tool in both directions. These saliency maps and heatmaps have potential but need more research. Overall, two general methods are used to explain how AI is making a prediction from an image. With feature attribution, the question is "Which pixels contribute most to the given prediction?" With counterfactuals, the question is "What pixels need to change to yield a different predictor?"

PRINCIPLE 132 • By learning from past mistakes and with more rigor, interpretation of mammograms can be significantly improved with machine learning methods.

The current approach of using mammogram data to improve patient outcomes is less than optimal, so AI is primarily needed because there is wide human variation.[9]

High-quality prospective imaging data sets from multiple institutions are needed for robust external validation studies of mammogram AI. These data sets must include a diverse population reflecting the population screened and should avoid being enriched with data sets (eg, mammograms that are 50% with and without breast cancer).

Although there are exciting advances in AI imaging, the question is "How can AI tools be implemented into practice?" Perhaps AI can start as a backup for radiologists, flagging mammograms that it predicts include cancer but were missed by the radiologist. "Please double-check this one." Ideally, this is performed as a pragmatic trial to ensure that it is safe and effective.

If the AI tool can detect cancer before the radiologist, the patient outcomes would certainly be improved, impacting many areas for further research. Do not ask "Can AI detect breast cancer as well as a radiologist?" rather "Can AI detect breast cancer on the mammogram a year earlier than the radiologist?" That would be a game-changer. Once detected, lymph node involvement is another promising area of AI imaging research for pathologists.

McKinney et al[10] described "an artificial intelligence (AI) system that is capable of surpassing human experts in breast cancer prediction." A pragmatic randomized controlled trial of a radiologist in usual care vs a radiologist in usual care plus an AI system that provides clinical decision support is the right strategy and the primary end point needs to be a composite outcome of survival and quality of life. Studies that simply show a better area under the receiver-operating-characteristic curve are a step in the right direction, but progress needs to continue with clinical implementation. Of course, there are major challenges—conducting such a study would require a large sample size and long-term outcomes. Having complete and accurate long-term outcome follow-up data for large populations is the current challenge.

PRINCIPLE 133 • Democratize expertise. AI will be used as clinical decision support in the United States, but in some countries, AI may be the only option.

Here are some facts about the shortage of specialists:

In China there is 1 radiologist for every 40,000 people[11] vs 11,000 in the United States.

In India there is 1 pathologist for every 9 million people vs 25,000 in the United States

In India there is 1 radiologist for every 100,000 people vs 11,000 in the United States.

In India there is a shortage of 127,000 eye doctors.

Machine learning methods are producing impressive results interpreting electrocardiograms

Machine learning methods have great potential in the interpretation of electrocardiograms (ECGs). Convolutional neural networks are often used due to the longitudinal structure of the image and have been able to make certain diagnoses, such as low ejection fraction, that cardiologists were unable to make, based on the ECG alone.[12] These systems may help save lives and help to triage work for cardiologists saving them time to focus on what is most important. More research is needed but AI-ECGs have the potential to predict atrial fibrillation, stroke, and acute myocardial infarction.

Using AI for retinal imaging has great potential not only for diabetic retinopathy but for many other health conditions.

Lily Peng and her group at Google Health have conducted some impressive research in this area. They have demonstrated that a deep learning algorithm had high sensitivity and specificity for detecting diabetic retinopathy.[13] Retinal scans can provide easy noninvasive ways to measure/screen for non-eye issues, such as cardiovascular health.

FOR MORE INFORMATION

MIT OpenCourseWare. Machine Learning for Healthcare. Lecture 25. Interpretability. Peter Szolovits.[14]
DeepMind × UCL Lecture 4/12. Advanced models for computer vision.
https://www.youtube.com/watch?v=_aUq7lmMfxo.
AI and the Future of Breast Cancer Detection and Risk Prediction— Constance Lehman, MD, PhD.[9]
https://www.youtube.com/watch?v=sboje1e2EJE.
Optimizing risk-based breast cancer screening policies with reinforcement learning. Adam Yala.[15]

CHAPTER SUMMARY

Since 2010, the annual ImageNet competitions have had teams compete to identify images from a database of 14 million pictures. This has led to numerous advances in deep learning that have been applied to medical imaging. Health care needs similar competitions to push researchers to improve against rigorous benchmarks. Multicenter imaging competitions are one way to promote data sharing to move this field forward with diverse populations.

High-quality prospective imaging data sets from multiple institutions are needed for robust external validation studies. These data sets must include a diverse population. Use data sets that represent the population and avoid enriched data sets (eg, mammograms that are 50% with and without breast cancer). The studies of AI in medical imaging need to follow modern reproducible research standards.

Deep learning methods have produced astounding results in medical imaging, but there are challenges in integrating these into practice and demonstrating value. As in all medicine, providing the clinician with a probability of a diagnosis from a medical image that is based on a black box remains a challenge. The probability must be accompanied with tools that explain the decision to the clinician and to help them explain it to the patient.

AI can assist radiologists and pathologists by prioritizing their worklist freeing up time to focus on the most important images. Although this may not seem as exciting as other applications, this is the type of AI tool that can add value and begin to build a symbiotic relationship between clinician and computer. To overcome resistance, AI tools could be introduced as a method of checking potentially missed diagnoses. If this works, it can open the way for the next phase of implementation research.

REFERENCES

1. Grimshaw JM, Eccles MP, Lavis JN, Hill SJ, Squires JE. Knowledge translation of research findings. *Implement Sci.* 2012;7:50.
2. Singh H, Meyer AN, Thomas EJ. The frequency of diagnostic errors in outpatient care: estimations from three large observational studies involving US adult populations. *BMJ Qual Saf.* 2014;23(9):727-731.
3. Krause J, Gulshan V, Rahimy E, et al. Grader variability and the importance of reference standards for evaluating machine learning models for diabetic retinopathy. *Ophthalmology.* 2018;125(8):1264-1272.
4. Elmore JG, Wells CK, Lee CH, et al. Variability in radiologists' interpretations of mammograms. *N Engl J Med.* 1994;331:1493-1499.
5. Elmore JG, Longton GM, Carney PA, et al. Diagnostic concordance among pathologists interpreting breast biopsy specimens. *JAMA.* 2015;313(11):1122-1132.
6. Jackson SL, Frederick PD, Pepe MS, et al. Diagnostic reproducibility: what happens when the same pathologist interprets the same breast biopsy specimen at two points in time?. *Ann Surg Oncol.* 2017;24(5):1234-1241.
7. Park SH, Han K. Methodologic guide for evaluating clinical performance and effect of artificial intelligence technology for medical diagnosis and prediction. *Radiology.* 2018;286(3):800-809.
8. Nagendran M, Chen Y, Lovejoy CA, et al. Artificial intelligence versus clinicians: systematic review of design, reporting standards, and claims of deep learning studies. *BMJ.* 2020;368:m689.
9. Lehman C. Artificial intelligence and the future of breast cancer detection and risk prediction. https://www.youtube.com/watch?v=sboje1e2EJE.
10. McKinney SM, Sieniek M, Godbole V, et al. International evaluation of an AI system for breast cancer screening. *Nature.* 2020;577(7788):89-94.
11. Gore JC. Artificial intelligence in medical imaging. *Magn Reson Imaging.* 2020;68:A1-A4.
12. Attia ZI, Noseworthy PA, Lopez-Jimenez F, et al. An artificial intelligence-enabled ECG algorithm for the identification of patients with atrial fibrillation during sinus rhythm: a retrospective analysis of outcome prediction. *Lancet.* 2019;394(10201):861-867.
13. Gulshan V, Peng L, Coram M, et al. Development and validation of a deep learning algorithm for detection of diabetic retinopathy in retinal fundus photographs. *JAMA.* 2016;316(22):2402-2410.
14. Szolovits P. MIT OpenCourseWare. Machine learning for healthcare. Lecture 25. Interpretability. https://www.youtube.com/watch?v=wDLzLN1tArA.
15. Yala A, Mikhael PG, Lehman C, et al. Optimizing risk-based breast cancer screening policies with reinforcement learning. *Nat Med.* 2022;28:136-143.

Pandemics—Using AI Tools to Improve Health Outcomes in a Pandemic

During the COVID-19 pandemic, we witnessed the remarkable and rapid biomedical success of the vaccine development, testing, and immunization and the remarkable work performed by dedicated health care professionals. AI tools and health care data, however, were not implemented in an optimal, modern way—but we can learn from this experience to improve for the future.

PRINCIPLE 134 • Health care infrastructure needs to develop nimble methods of collection and sharing of data.

Pulling COVID-19 data was like pulling teeth. The major bottleneck in applying AI during the COVID-19 pandemic was obtaining the correct data—in a timely way. Conditions were changing so rapidly and messaging was so varied and politically influenced that hospitals and government agencies were unable to share data in an optimal way. Clinical laboratories were reluctant to report important data, such as viral load. Even the Centers for Disease Control and Prevention (CDC) was not set up to share data at the speed at which it was needed. Health care systems were not prepared to rapidly collect new data, export it, build models, and implement models. Combined, these delays led to misinformation and poor outcomes. Enhanced data sharing solutions are a priority. The National Institutes of Health and the CDC should provide targeted funding to develop ways to nimbly collect and share this type of data.

To create a model to identify which patients should be screened, a data set similar to the one shown in Figure 18.1 is needed. Note: all identifiers can be removed from a data set for building these models. AI does not require personal health identifiers. The concerns about privacy can be addressed and then deidentified data sets can be used for models. Health care data privacy

case	contact	temperature	gender male	fever	bmi	age	anosmia	cancer	o2sat	covid19positive	poor_outcome	probability_covid	probability_poor_outcome
1	1	103.5	1	1	29.5	64	1	0	96	1	1	97.7	28.3
2	0	98.6	0	0	25.1	35	0	0	98	0	0	4.7	7.9
3	0	100.5	0	1	25.1	35	0	0	98	0	0	13.6	7.9
4	1	102.3	0	1	27.3	44	1	0	99	0	0	84.7	9.6

FIGURE 18.1. An example of a deidentified hypothetical data set that could be used for creating COVID-19 models. Note the last two columns are the probability results that are generated after building the model. These models do not need data sets that have protected health information.

issues are critically important, but there are solutions, and this should not become a complete obstacle to using data in a smarter way—especially when lives depend on it.

PRINCIPLE 135 • Develop, validate, and use diagnostic predictive models to identify who needs to be tested.

The process of deciding who needs COVID-19 testing has not been completely evidence based, and in the future, AI can be used to identify the people most likely to be infected to focus testing resources (Figure 18.2). Some AI applications like this require new information architecture for collecting information as it happened while being nimble enough to change rapidly. For example, anosmia (loss of smell) was not routinely collected on patients but became a valuable piece of information in predicting who was positive. The data that need to be collected change during a pandemic and with new variants. As patients are tested, they can be asked a few key questions that are stored electronically in a database and this information can be fed back to improve the models. Public health

Predictor Variables	Input Values		Coding	Coefficients	
Have you been in contact with someone who was confirmed or suspected of having Coronavirus/COVID-19?	1		0=no, 1=yes	1.12	
Have you had a fever in the past 2 weeks?	1		0=no, 1=yes	0.63	
Loss of smell (anosmia)	1		0=no, 1=yes	1.94	
Cough	0		0=no, 1=yes	0.46	
Temperature (F)	103.5			0.28	
Gender	0		0=female, 1=male	0.35	
Have you had a sore throat in the past 2 weeks?	0		0=no, 1=yes	−0.51	
Traveled long distance in the last month?	0		0=no, 1=yes	0.49	
Myalgia/Malaise (muscle pain)	0		0=no, 1=yes	0.42	
Model output:				−30.57	Intercept
Probability of a positive COVID-19 test (%)	88.6%		$1/(1+2.718^{-Z})$	2.05	Z value

FIGURE 18.2. A hypothetical predictive model of COVID-19 positivity. This example illustrates how a transparent predictive model can be used to the estimate the probability that a person would test positive for COVID-19. The Z value is simply the sum of the intercept and the input values multiplied by their coefficients. This Z value is plugged into the formula $((1/(1 + 2.718^{-Z}))$ × 100) to produce the probability of being positive for COVID-19.

officials will then be able to move away from an all-or-none approach (test everyone vs test no one) to one that uses a predictive model to compute probability of being positive.

The models also provide valuable information to public health officials. For example, in 2020, the models clearly showed that the symptom of sore throat actually decreased the probability of being positive for COVID-19.[1] Yet, public health officials continued to list sore throat as one of the symptoms, causing public confusion and inefficiencies in prioritizing testing.

PRINCIPLE 136 • Screening based on a dichotomized temperature was not as effective as using the continuous temperature in a full predictive model.

Screening for a temperature greater than or equal to 100.4 F as a sign of COVID-19 was an ineffective approach, but this is a good example of how a receiver-operating-characteristic (ROC) curve can be used to compare various approaches. See Chapter 3 for more about ROC curves. If there is no risk stratification, the area under the receiver-operating-characteristic curve (AUC) is 0.5, by using a temperature check of ≥100.4 F, the AUC improved only slightly to 0.52. Using the continuous temperature would provide an AUC of 0.63, but using a simple predictive model of temperature, with gender, loss of smell, cough, and muscle pain, etc, would improve this to 0.70. Although not perfect, an improvement over the current practice can add value. Also, note the information wasted by dichotomizing temperature (the AUC dropped from 0.63 to 0.52).

Optimal cut points and prognostic thresholds (such as a temperature ≥100.4 F) are outdated approaches and rarely replicate, so instead use the continuous predictor and outcome probability. If an optimal cut point on an ROC curve must be calculated, there are a few options. The "elbow" of the ROC is statistically the optimal cut point to maximize sensitivity and specificity. The Youden index can identify the exact point. The cut point of ≥100.4 F has a sensitivity of 6.2% and a specificity of 97.4%. This means that 93.8% of the people positive for COVID-19 pass this screening test (Figure 18.3). Although these are complex issues, the bottom line is that a continuous temperature combined with other factors would provide better risk stratification. Screening models can be implemented at points were there are temperature checks simply by having a computer screen that captures the additional questions and compute risk of COVID-19.

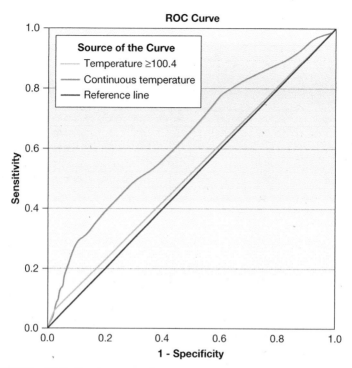

FIGURE 18.3. Receiver-operating-characteristic curve of screening for COVID-19 with a dichotomized temperature vs a continuous temperature. Using a continuous temperature provides an area under the receiver-operating-characteristic curve (AUC) of 0.63, but dichotomizing the temperature reduces the AUC to 0.52, which is close to useless.

PRINCIPLE 137 • Among people who test positive, develop, validate, automate, and use prognostic predictive models for the probability of poor outcome.

A key question that is best answered with predictive models is: "Among those who test positive for COVID-19, what is the probability that the person will have poor outcome (require ICU care, require ventilator support, or die)?" This can be accomplished with a logistic regression model of easy to obtain variables, such as age, gender, cancer patient, oxygen saturation, diabetes, body mass index, and white blood cell count (Figure 18.4). If any of these are missing, substituting the median value performs well. Combining

Predictor Variables	Input Values		Coding	Coefficients	
Age	92			0.02	
Gender	1		0 = Female, 1 = Male	0.61	
Cancer patient	1		0 = No, 1 = Yes	0.92	
O_2 saturation	92			−0.14	
Diabetes	1		0 = No, 1 = Yes	0.45	
BMI	29.1			0.03	
WBC	6.8			0.04	
Model output:				10.12	Intercept
Predicted Risk of Ventilator, ICU, or Death	81.8%		$1/(1+2.718^{-Z})$	1.51	Z Value

FIGURE 18.4. A hypothetical predictive model of poor outcome for patients who test positive for COVID-19. This example illustrates how a transparent predictive model can be used to estimate the probability of poor outcomes among patients who are positive for COVID-19. The Z value is simply the sum of the intercept and the input values multiplied by their coefficients. This Z value is plugged into the formula $((1/(1 + 2.718^{-Z})) \times 100)$ to produce the probability of poor outcome. BMI, body mass index; WBC, white blood cell count.

these variables provides an accurate estimate of which patients are likely to have a poor outcome. Models such as this can be used to identify high-risk patients early and enroll them in prevention protocols. The high-risk patients can also be provided with treatments and increased surveillance. Many of the COVID-19 treatment studies struggled to identify these patients in a timely way. So, what needs to be changed to implement these models? Health care leaders need to understand how the models can help them accomplish their goals. Then they need to mobilize the fragmented resources to collect the right data, create the models, implement the models, and develop an effector arm.

The prognostic models can be used to prioritize the order of vaccination to ensure that the people who are most likely to have poor outcome, if infected, get immunized first.

When the various vaccines were being distributed, there was a missed opportunity to randomize them. This would have provided valuable needed data on the comparative effectiveness. It would have been easy to ask people "Would you like the Pfizer or Moderna vaccine? Or would it be OK if we select at random so that we can improve the science?"

Chapter 18 • Pandemics

Specific models need to be developed for children

We found that the factors that predicted poor outcome among children with COVID-19 were very different from adults. Therefore, we created and published a paper on a predictive model specifically for pediatric patients.[1] Since the variants change during a pandemic, these models need to be updated during the course of a pandemic. Collecting the right data, designing, and implementing a new model is extremely challenging, particularly when the health care system is stretched to its limits.

COVID-19 vaccine research in children was delayed by the mistaken notion that we protect children by not randomizing them at the same time as the adults. Children need more rigorous evidence to protect them—not less.

PRINCIPLE 138 • Forward-thinking health care leaders will be supportive of using predictive models and prepared to implement them in the workflow.

An obvious challenge during the COVID-19 pandemic was that our current health care system was not prepared to implement AI models since there is no process to insert a model into the workflow. Many were comfortable to continue screening in an old-fashioned way, such as with a dichotomized temperature, which was pure theater. We need to educate future medical leaders about how models work and how they can be implemented in practice. There are deep problems with the antiquated health systems in the United States that became apparent during the COVID-19 pandemic. Those who work to create and implement AI tools are often paralyzed by the bureaucracy of our health care system.

Our health care system should have periodic pandemic "fire drills" to become efficient at collecting, sharing data, and implementing AI tools. This preparedness will probably need to be led by the Joint Commission, OSHA, the CDC, or the NIH. This change will not happen without strong leadership. The groups can also provide funding for solutions, such as federated learning. The groups can also join forces to create deidentified data sets for AI competitions with clear benchmarks.

i FOR MORE INFORMATION

COVID-19 Positive Risk of Severe COVID-19. Michael Kattan.[2,3]
Prediction models for diagnosis and prognosis of COVID-19: systematic review and critical appraisal. Laure Wynats et al[4]

CHAPTER SUMMARY

AI models are needed for precise risk stratification in medicine, in general, but more urgently in public health. Without this risk stratification, the all-or-none policy creates more problems. Our health care system needs to be prepared to build, implement, and embrace AI tools in a timely way for pandemics and other emergency situations. AI technology is needed to detect the earliest signs of a pandemic as well as the spread. Tools to risk stratify people to prioritize testing are also essential to the control of a pandemic. Of those who are found positive for the virus, the AI tools are vital to providing risk stratification for probability of poor outcomes. Finally, AI can be valuable is distributing the vaccine in the most efficient manner. By understanding the pain points that AI researchers encountered with the COVID-19 pandemic, we can learn lessons to remove these barriers so that we are prepared to use the power of AI for the future in many ways.

REFERENCES

1. Howard LM, Garguilo K, Gillon J, et al. The first 1000 symptomatic pediatric SARS-CoV-2 infections in an integrated health care system: a prospective cohort study. *BMC Pediatr.* 2021;21(1):403.
2. Kattan M. COVID-19 Positive risk of severe COVID-19. https://riskcalc.org/SevereCOVID19/
3. Jehi L, Ji X, Milinovich A, et al. Individualizing risk prediction for positive coronavirus disease 2019 testing: results from 11,672 patients. *Chest.* 2020;158(4):1364-1375.
4. Wynants L, Van Calster B, Collins GS, et al. Prediction models for diagnosis and prognosis of covid-19: systematic review and critical appraisal. *BMJ.* 2020;369:m1328. Update in: *BMJ.* 2021;372:n236. Erratum in: *BMJ.* 2020;369:m2204.

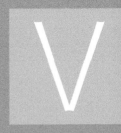

The Future

19

Careers—How to Build a Career Around AI in Medicine by Turning This Playbook Into a Reality

"Before we work on artificial intelligence why don't we do something about natural stupidity?"

—A JOKE BY THE COMPUTER SCIENTIST, STEVE POLYAK.

PRINCIPLE 139 • **AI will displace some jobs in health care, but it will also create new high-paying, rewarding jobs. The key is to develop the skills for the new AI roles.**

The impact of Artificial Intelligence (AI) on the job market will be similar to what happened as the result of personal computers and the Internet—technology eliminated automatable jobs but created many new careers that were often superior—but only for those who changed and developed modern skills.

"Change before you have to."

—JACK WELCH.

AI will certainly result in some worker displacement in health care, particularly for those who have a job that is highly repetitive or involves prediction/classification that could be performed more accurately and precisely by an AI tool. Although AI will not replace doctors, doctors who learn AI skills will advance their careers faster than those who do not. Since approximately 94% of physicians say they do not know enough about AI, developing a general understanding of AI, and particularly AI implementation skills, is a smart career move. The same applies to nurses and health care administrators, managers, executives, and biostatisticians. This will be a gradual change—but it will happen. Job displacement is a fact of life and will not be stopped by AI critics or data activists.

Each year in the United States, more than $10 billion is invested in health care AI and there is a shortage of qualified people to fill these jobs (Table 19.1). If you are a student aiming for a job in AI in medicine, focus on the right course load (Table 19.2) while aggressively teaching yourself about AI and AI programming in your spare time. If you already have a job

TABLE 19.1   In-Demand AI Jobs in Health Care

Job Title

Data scientist
Senior software engineer
Machine learning engineer
Data engineer
Director of analytics
Principal scientist
Software engineer
Computer vision engineer
Software developer
Software architect
Principal software engineer
AI data scientist
Biostatistician/statistician
Computer scientist
Health informatics specialist
Clinical informatics analyst
Research engineer
Big data engineer/architect
AI research scientist
AI architect
Deep learning engineer
Robotics engineer
Data analyst
Algorithm engineer

TABLE 19.2	Courses to Take to Qualify for a Career in AI and for Admission to Graduate School for AI

Programming course in Python
TensorFlow
Data analysis
Computer science
R programming
Three semesters of college calculus (through multivariable calculus)
Linear algebra
Statistics and biostatistics
JavaScript
Biology and human anatomy/physiology
Genetics
Graphics
Data science
Machine learning in health care
Deep learning
Medical writing
Communication skills in general

and are looking to transition into AI, you can focus on your self-education and personal branding. Consider going back to school to earn an advanced degree in AI or a related field. Most well-paying AI jobs in medicine require an advanced degree. Approximately 63% of data scientists have a graduate degree (48% master's degree, 15% doctoral degree).[1] Kaggle, a Google company with an active online community of data scientists, offers data sets, resources, and competitions for machine learning practitioners. According to the 2021 Kaggle survey, only 16% of data scientists are women.[1] So, there are great opportunities for women who want to enter this field, as many employers will be working to adjust this imbalance.

PRINCIPLE 140 • **Earn a degree in AI, computer science, biostatistics, biomedical informatics, engineering, biology, mathematics, information management, or a related field. Since there is a shortage of AI talent, AI companies and start-ups will be hiring from a broad range of related areas.**

Go as far as you can with your formal education and consider a combination of degrees or majors that will be marketable (Table 19.3). For example, a bachelor's degree in biology and a master's degree in biostatistics, or a dual major of genetics and computer science. Any combination of analytics plus biomedical science will be valuable. Most professional AI job skills and knowledge are learned after formal schooling is completed, but the formal education and degrees open doors that are otherwise shut.

For an example of an application process for a graduate program in biostatistics, see the Vanderbilt Biostatistics website: https://www.vanderbilt.edu/biostatistics-graduate/application-process/ and the Biomedical Informatics website: https://medschool.vanderbilt.edu/biomedical-informatics/research-ms-and-phd-program/.

Avoid predatory short-term training programs in data science that are expensive but lightweight.

Amassing student debt from a program that does not prepare you for an actual AI career is unwise. More and more of these expensive bootcamps and for-profit intensive training programs will take your money but fail to properly prepare you for employment. They teach gimmicks, such as word clouds rather than actual job skills with a solid foundation. Be sure the program teaches how to create and evaluate statistical models as well as neural

TABLE 19.3	A Sample of High-Quality AI Programs in the United States

California Institute of Technology
Carnegie Mellon University
Columbia University
Cornell University
Georgia Institute of Technology
Harvard University
Massachusetts Institute of Technology
Stanford University
University of California—Berkeley
University of Illinois—Urbana-Champaign
University of Texas—Austin
University of Washington
Yale University

networks. Many of these new data science training programs need to bring science to data science before they are worth an investment of your time or money.

PRINCIPLE 141 • Self-education in AI is your key to success.

Understand how to analyze data and learn the theory as well as the mechanics of AI and statistics. See Table 16.1 in "Publishing Your Medical Research"[2] for a list of the most commonly used inferential statistical techniques in modern medical research. Start at the top of this list and master each method. The statistical flowchart in "Publishing Your Medical Research" will guide you as you learn these tools.[2]

If you are not interested in more formal schooling or are unable to invest the time and money in these education programs, you can still find a high-paying job in AI in medicine, but it will be a challenge to get your foot in the door and you must work extra hard at developing your skills and branding yourself.

Your formal education will not completely prepare you for a job in AI; you must be aggressive in your self-education. Fortunately, it is possible to teach yourself many of the skills that are important in AI. First step, read the books in Table 19.4 and learn the in-demand programming languages in Table 19.5.

Use publicly available medical data sets to polish your AI skills:
Stanford's AIMI (Artificial Intelligence in Medicine & Imaging) center—a free repository of imaging datasets for researchers.
https://aimi.stanford.edu/shared-datasets
https://hai.stanford.edu/news/open-source-movement-comes-medical-datasets
iMerit—an AI data solutions company with a website of "20 Free Life Sciences, Healthcare, and Medical Datasets for Machine Learning".
https://imerit.net/blog/20-free-life-sciences-healthcare-and-medical-datasets-for-machine-learning-all-pbm/
MNIST database—Modified National Institute of Standards and Technology database is a large database of handwritten digits. This can be used to practice creating a neural network.
http://yann.lecun.com/exdb/mnist/
Kaggle—"Top medical datasets."
https://www.kaggle.com/general/168211.

Interactive development environments to master

An interactive development environment (IDE) is a software tool with a graphical user interface and a text editor to write and compile code to make it easier for computer programmers to develop software.

TABLE 19.4	AI Books to Read—The "No Doctor Left Behind" Reading List

Deep Medicine. Eric Topol.[3]

Thinking, Fast and Slow. Daniel Kahneman.[4]

Clinical Prediction Models—A Practical Approach to Development, Validation, and Updating. Ewout Steyerberg.[5]

Publishing Your Medical Research. Daniel Byrne.[2]
https://www.slideshare.net/DanielByrne12/
publishing-your-medical-research-125452257

Artificial Intelligence: The Insights You Need from Harvard Business Review. Thomas Davenport, Erik Brynjolfsson, Andrew McAfee, H. James Wilson.[6]

AI Superpowers: China, Silicon Valley, And The New World Order. Kai-Fu Lee.[7]

The Ethical Algorithm: The Science of Socially Aware Algorithm Design. Michael Kearns, Aaron Roth et al[8]

Hands-On Machine Learning with Scikit-Learn, Keras, and TensorFlow: Concepts, Tools, and Techniques to Build Intelligent Systems. Aurélien Géron.[9]

Deep Learning with Python. François Chollet.[10]

The Hundred-Page Machine Learning Book. Andriy Burkov.[11]

Machine Learning: An Algorithmic Perspective. Stephen Marsland.[12]

An Introduction to Statistical Learning: with Applications in R. Gareth James, Daniela Witten, Trevor Hastie, Robert Tibshirani.[13]

Python for Data Analysis: Data Wrangling with Pandas, NumPy, and IPython. Wes McKinney.[14]

Machine Learning: A Probabilistic Perspective. Kevin Murphy.[15]

Practical Statistics for Data Scientists: 50+ Essential Concepts Using R and Python. Peter Bruce Andrew Bruce, Peter Gedeck.[16]

Reinforcement Learning: An Introduction. Richard S. Sutton and Andrew G. Barto. (The book is freely available here: http://incompleteideas.net/book/RLbook2020.pdf)[17]

Statistical Modeling for Biomedical Researchers: A Simple Introduction to the Analysis of Complex Data. William D. Dupont.[18]

Encyclopedia of Biostatistics. Armitage P, Colton T.

TABLE 19.5	Learn the In-demand Programming Languages, Packages, Libraries

Name	Description
SciKit-Learn	Open-source machine learning library for Python programming. 82% of data scientists use SciKit-Learn.
https://scikit-learn.org	
Python	One of the most popular high-level programming languages in AI.
https://www.python.org/	
TensorFlow	A popular, free, open-source platform for training machine learning models. Google developed these open-source deep learning tools. TensorFlow makes it easy to specify a neural network and train a model. A Neural Network Playground—TensorFlow: https://playground.tensorflow.org
https://www.tensorflow.org/	
R and RStudio	Open-source statistical computing and graphical software and GUI.
https://www.r-project.org/ https://www.rstudio.com/	
JavaScript	A programming language that is used for most websites.
https://www.javascript.com/	
Keras	An open-source neural network software library providing high-level APIs. Keras acts as an interface for the TensorFlow library.
https://www.python.org/	
Java	A widely used AI programming language.
https://www.java.com/en/	

(Continued)

TABLE 19.5	*Continued*

Name	Description
PyTorch https://pytorch.org/	For visual and natural language processing.
C++ https://en.wikipedia.org/wiki/C%2B%2B	A very fast AI programming language used for robotics and speech.
SQL https://en.wikipedia.org/wiki/SQL	"Sequel" (Structured Query Language) used in programming and designed for managing data
Scala https://www.scala-lang.org/	Object-oriented and functional programming in one concise, high-level language.

Commonly used IDEs include Jupyter Notebook, Visual Studio Code (VSCode), JupyterLab, PyCharm, RStudio, Eclipse, and Android Studio.

Master a statistical software package such as R, Stata, or IBM SPSS

The most commonly used statistical software packages in medicine are SAS, R, Stata, and IBM SPSS.[2] SAS, Stata, and IBM SPSS are commercial packages. R and RStudio are free, open-source, and can be downloaded from these sites: https://www.r-project.org/ and https://www.rstudio.com/.

PRINCIPLE 142 • Throughout your career have a 5-year plan. Focus on becoming the expert at the skills needed "5 years down the road."

Since AI and medicine are overwhelmingly complex fields, you must clearly identify what you need to learn that will be most important in obtaining your first, or next, job. Then you must break this into small skills that you can master. If you break down your skills into something very specific, you can become skilled at something very quickly. For example, within 1 week you could develop a high level of expertise in creating classification and regression trees with the rpart package in R (https://cran.r-project.org/web/packages/rpart/rpart.pdf). This might take 40 to 50 hours of practice and study, but it is very doable and this is a marketable AI skill. Then continue learning the next most important skill. Develop a unique niche with skills that employers are looking for. Your mentors can guide you.

PRINCIPLE 143 • **Take advantage of the wealth of free online AI education programs (Table 19.6).**

TABLE 19.6	Online Courses and Videos

1. Coursera—Deep Learning Specialization. Andrew Ng.
   https://www.coursera.org/specializations/deep-learning
2. MIT Introduction to Deep Learning 6.S191. Alexander Amini.
   https://www.youtube.com/watch?v=njKP3FqW3Sk
3. MIT Machine Learning for Healthcare 6.S897. David Sontag.
   https://www.youtube.com/watch?v=vof7x8r_ZUA
4. Introduction to Machine Learning and AI. Thore Graepel.
   https://www.youtube.com/watch?v=7R52wiUgxZl
5. The Deep Learning Lectures Series. DeepMind × UCL.
   https://deepmind.com/learning-resources/
       deep-learning-lecture-series-2020
6. Kaggle Learn Courses.
   https://www.kaggle.com/learn
7. Udemy.
   https://www.udemy.com/
8. DataCamp.
   https://www.datacamp.com/
9. DataCamp for R.
   https://www.datacamp.com/courses/free-introduction-to-r
10. Udacity.
    https://www.udacity.com/
11. Data Science Bits. The Definitive Guide to F1 Score. Filipe Penha.
    https://www.youtube.com/watch?v=_OCYto4zK0g
12. AlphaGo—The Movie.
    https://www.youtube.com/watch?v=WXuK6gekU1Y

(Continued)

TABLE 19.6 *Continued*

13. StatQuest, Josh Starmer.
https://www.youtube.com/watch?v=CqOfi41LfDw
14. 3Blue1Brown.
https://www.youtube.com/watch?v=aircAruvnKk
15. Edureka! AI in Healthcare.
https://www.youtube.com/watch?v=j6EB9HO6acE
16. CrashCourse. Artificial Intelligence.
https://www.youtube.com/playlist?list=
PL8dPuuaLjXtO65LeD2p4_Sb5XQ51par_b
17. OpenAI. Machine Learning For Medical Image Analysis—How It Works.
https://www.youtube.com/watch?v=VKnoyiNxflk
18. Lex Fridman podcasts.
https://www.youtube.com/watch?v=UwwBG-MbniY
19. Khan Academy. Salman Khan.
https://www.khanacademy.org/computing/computer-science
20. SimpliLearn. How To Become An Artificial Intelligence Engineer.
https://www.youtube.com/watch?v=uBV0w8Qwhv4
21. The 7 Steps of ML—Google Developers.
https://www.youtube.com/watch?v=nKW8Ndu7Mjw
22. In the age of AI—Frontline PBS YouTube.
https://www.youtube.com/watch?v=5dZ_lvDgevk
23. CodeEmporium.
https://www.youtube.com/watch?v=9E-Isou160g
24. AI and Deep Learning—Two Minute Papers.
https://www.youtube.com/watch?v=Lu56xVIZ40M&list=PLujx
SBD-JXglGL3ERdDOhthD3jTlfudC2
25. TechCrunch.
https://www.youtube.com/watch?v=jiXwXg2CUWM
26. Reinforcement Learning online course (13 lectures) by Hado van Hasselt. DeepMind x UCL.
https://www.youtube.com/watch?v=TCCjZe0y4Qc
27. Getting Started with R. Mike Marin.
https://www.youtube.com/watch?v=riONFzJdXcs&list=PLq
zoL9-eJTNARFXxgwbqGo56NtbJnB37A
28. Data management for clinical research. REDCap. Paul Harris.
https://www.coursera.org/instructor/~1347429

PRINCIPLE 144 • Create a personal branding to advance your career in AI.

Medicine and AI are huge fields with busy people doing the hiring. You must clearly define where your expertise lies, along with your combinations of skills, experience, and personality. Differentiate yourself from the other job candidates. Google your own name and keep improving yourself until you are happy with your personal branding (Table 19.7).

Customize your resume for the AI career you desire

If you are applying for jobs in academia, also create a CV (curriculum vitae), which is a longer and more detailed version of your resume. Improve your education and experience to honestly build your resume to match one of the high-paying jobs as given in Table 19.1. Tailor your resume for the job and ask for plenty of feedback before you send it. Make it very clear that you meet the criteria for the posted job description. Include an objective statement. According to an eye-tracking study,[19] recruiters spend ~7 seconds per resume. So, make it easy for them to see that you are the most qualified person to interview. Highlight your data analysis skills, experience with software development, and experience with various programs such as Python and R. Document on your resume that you have excellent data management skills. Many people hiring will be looking for someone who can perform data wrangling work for them. These are good entry-level jobs to accept as you master more advanced skills. Find a copy of the resume of the person who has the job you want. Keep improving your education, skills, and experience until your resume looks like the example.

Improve your communication skills and become fluently bilingual in AI and medicine. If you enjoy teaching, collaborating in teams, and have strong communication skills, highlight that on your resume because these skills are often lacking in candidates.

In addition to technical and coding skills, work on developing the ability to understand health care terminology, human anatomy, workflow, and the business aspects of medicine. To be successful and earn a good salary, you must understand not only the technical aspects but also the larger issues and the clinical subject matter. Otherwise, you will be a poorly paid programmer doing uninteresting work.

PRINCIPLE 145 • Attend and participate in AI conferences and job fairs.

One way to find a job in AI is to submit an abstract to a conference (Table 19.8). Abstracts for posters have a high rate of acceptance, and this will

TABLE 19.7	Resources for Personal Branding for AI Careers

GitHub—a platform for building, sharing, and showcasing your code and software.
https://github.com/
Kaggle—an online community for AI, with data sets, competitions, and education.
https://www.kagglc.com/
LinkedIn—a platform for professional networking and job searches.
https://www.linkedin.com
Google Scholar—an easy to set up platform that organizes your scholarly publications allows you to customize your profile.
https://scholar.google.com/
Your personal web page—Anyone looking to advance their career in AI should create their own web page. Post your job talk here.
Twitter—a microblogging and networking service useful for your visibility and branding.
https://twitter.com
ResearchGate—a networking site for scientists and researchers to share publications and find collaborators.
https://www.researchgate.net/
Google Knowledge Panel—the information box that appears to the right of a Google search. You can customize your own knowledge panel by following these instructions:
https://support.google.com/knowledgepanel/answer/7534842
ArXiv—pronounced "archive"—(the X is the Greek letter chi). Open-access archive for scholarly articles often used by AI researchers.
https://arxiv.org/
YouTube—the online video sharing platform.
https://www.youtube.com
https://www.youtube.com/watch?v=s3B7OeEHGRo

allow you to meet potential hiring managers. See "Publishing Your Medical Research" for more information on writing abstracts.

PRINCIPLE 146 • Find multiple AI mentors who will help you advance your career.

TABLE 19.8	AI Conferences

AMIA (American Medical Informatics Association) Annual
  Symposium
  https://amia.org/education-events/annual-symposium
The International Conference on Learning Representations
  https://iclr.cc/
International Conference on Artificial Intelligence in Medicine.
  https://aime23.aimedicine.info/
JSM (Joint Statistical Meeting)
  https://ww2.amstat.org/meetings/jsm/2023/
AIMED—The Global Summit.
  https://ai-med.io/all-events/global-summits/aimed-22/
NIPS Conference on Neural Information Processing Systems
  https://videos.neurips.cc/
EmTech Digital—MIT Technology Review's annual event on AI
  redefINE Event 2021
  https://www.youtube.com/watch?v=HgZBqoLAH-
    j0&list=PL3UpcvaDU_FkmNdfYR3x3VNW0FUVo0ZH-
    &index=3

One of the most important steps to take is to find the right mentors who will invest time in you. First you need to find mentors who can really teach you something valuable. Second you need to find a way to provide value to them. These are busy people and will not want to spend time mentoring you unless you solve an important problem for them or bring them some value. Do not rely on one mentor; it is better to have a team of mini-mentors who teach in different ways. Quora, the question-and-answer website (https://www.quora.com/), can function as another form of mentoring.

PRINCIPLE 147 • Create a start-up or become a self-employed AI consultant.

When ready, consider starting a consulting business on the side that specializes in AI and then gradually build up your portfolio of clients. Although this might take several years, a gradual shift from a salaried to self-employed income will make your chance of success much greater. If you decide to become a full-time entrepreneur, be sure not to burn any bridges when you leave your job. Instead convert your former employer into a consulting client with a retainer agreement.

AI start-ups and vendors looking for business in health care should partner with an academic medical center to assess implementation with randomization. To improve your odds of success as an AI entrepreneur, scope the project carefully and then form a team with a physician-scientist as the principal investigator. Although this will be uncomfortable for some entrepreneurs, tone down the hype and embrace randomization to focus on improving patient outcomes. This approach, although more difficult in the short term, will give you the competitive long-term edge. To convince hospital leaders to invest in an AI tool, you need to convince them that the return on investment will be impressive; convincing them that they will break even is not sufficient.

Be savvy about applying for AI grants

The National Institutes of Health has an annual budget of more than $43 billion. Patient-Centered Outcomes Research Institute has an annual budget of more than $300 million. Physician-scientists are successfully winning AI grants from these, and other sources and the principles in this book will help with a competitive grant application. Good grantsmanship requires writing these grants in a way that is rigorous and objective regarding model building techniques and philosophies. Therefore, propose an agnostic approach by developing and evaluating both machine learning and logistic regression to satisfy the reviewers. Grant reviewers are smart and experienced. Attempts to bamboozle them with complexity or jargon will result in rejection. Since many reviewers understand that the literature is full of unused models, you will want to propose a pragmatic trial to assess impact.

AI Researchers Portal. https://www.ai.gov/ai-researchers-portal/

This website provides a wealth of information about federal resources to help with your AI project. The portal provides searchable repositories of federal grant programs relevant to AI and a wide variety of data and computing resources useful for AI research.

AI.gov—The National AI Initiative. https://www.ai.gov/

TABLE 19.9	10 Rules for a Successful Implementation of Health Care AI

1. Be realistic about how hard it will be to integrate AI into health care.
2. Address the concerns about using AI in health care.
3. Improve the level of teamwork among groups that do not normally work together.
4. Help all involved become comfortable with randomization.
5. Focus on improving health outcomes that are important to patients.
6. Change the financial and career promotion incentives for the team so that they align with using AI to improve health outcomes.
7. Keep an open mind about various AI techniques and avoid falling in love with one method.
8. Raise the standards with rigorous evaluations regarding a successful implementation of AI.
9. Hire excellent project managers to create forward progress and avoid Brownian motion that can stall these projects.
10. Put the physician-scientists in front and have marketing and salespeople limit their claims to what researchers have proven—replace hyperbole with science.

 FOR MORE INFORMATION

How to get a job in machine learning without a degree. Karolina Sowinska.[20]
AI Career Pathways: Put Yourself on the Right Track. Workera[21]

CHAPTER SUMMARY

Have a clear plan for your career and the skills necessary for your dream job. Spend at least 1 hour per day learning how to code. Spend several hours per day reading and studying in a very focused way to master the next most important skill.

The work in AI in health care today is at a profound level but needs smart people to take it to the next level to improve health outcomes and successful health care leaders will provide broad AI training for their employees to help them accomplish this transformation into the age of AI implementation.

We began this book with the big unanswered question: "**Can Artificial Intelligence be used to improve patient outcomes?**" As you can see from the examples and information in this book, the answer is YES, but one must follow these principles and avoid short cuts (Table 19.9). By doing so, it is possible to turn this blueprint into a reality to improve health outcomes.

REFERENCES

1. Kaggle's. *State of Data Science and Machine Learning Survey!* 2021. https://www.kaggle.com/kaggle-survey-2021

2. Byrne. *Publishing Your Medical Research.* Wolters Kluwer; 2017. https://www.slideshare.net/DanielByrne12/publishing-your-medical-research-125452257

3. Topol E. *Deep Medicine: How Artificial Intelligence Can Make Healthcare Human Again.* Basic Books; 2019.

4. Kahneman D. *Thinking, Fast and Slow.* Farrar, Straus and Giroux; 2011.

5. Steyerberg EW. *Clinical Prediction Models—A Practical Approach to Development, Validation, and Updating.* Springer; 2019.

6. Davenport T, Brynjolfsson E, McAfee A, James Wilson H. *Artificial Intelligence: The Insights You Need From Harvard Business Review.* Harvard Business Review Press; 2019.

7. Lee K-F. *AI Superpowers: China, Silicon Valley, and the New World Order.* Mariner Books; 2018.

8. Kearns M, Roth A. *The Ethical Algorithm: The Science of Socially Aware Algorithm Design.* Oxford University Press; 2019.

9. Géron A. *Hands-On Machine Learning with Scikit-Learn, Keras, and TensorFlow: Concepts, Tools, and Techniques to Build Intelligent Systems.* O'Reilly Media, Inc.; 2019.

10. Chollet F. *Deep Learning with Python.* Manning Publications; 2017.

11. Burkov A. *The Hundred-Page Machine Learning Book.* Andriy Burkov; 2019.

12. Marsland S. *Machine Learning: An Algorithmic Perspective.* CRC Press; 2014.

13. James G, Witten D, Hastie T, Tibshirani R. *An Introduction to Statistical Learning: With Applications in R.* Springer; 2021.

14. McKinney W. *Python for Data Analysis: Data Wrangling with Pandas, NumPy, and IPython.* O'Reilly Media, Inc.; 2017.
15. Murphy K. *Machine Learning: A Probabilistic Perspective.* MIT Press; 2012.
16. Bruce P, Bruce A, Gedeck P. *Practical Statistics for Data Scientists: 50+ Essential Concepts Using R and Python.* O'Reilly Media, Inc.; 2020.
17. Sutton RS, Barto AG. *Reinforcement Learning: An Introduction.* The book is freely available here: http://incompleteideas.net/book/RLbook2020.pdf.
18. Dupont WD. *Statistical Modeling for Biomedical Researchers: A Simple Introduction to the Analysis of Complex Data.* Accessed September 22, 2022. https://doi.org/10.1017/CBO9780511575884.002
19. Ladders. *Eye-Tracking Study.* 2018. https://www.theladders.com/static/images/basicSite/pdfs/TheLadders-EyeTracking-StudyC2.pdf
20. Sowinska K. How to get a job in MACHINE LEARNING without a DEGREE. https://www.youtube.com/watch?v=ZPXh_-_iHR8.
21. Workera. AI career pathways: put yourself on the right track. https://workera.ai/resource_downloads/ai_career_pathways/

Index

Note: Page numbers followed by "f" indicate figures and "t" indicate tables.